HAVING LEUKEMIA ISN'T SO BAD. OF COURSE IT WOULDN'T BE MY FIRST CHOICE.

A Story of Hope for Families of Children with Cancer

by

Cynthia Krumme

Sargasso Enterprises
14 Wildwood Street
Winchester, MA 01890

Although the author and publisher have made every effort to ensure the accuracy and completeness of information contained in this book, we assume no responsibility for errors, inaccuracies, omissions, or any inconsistency herein. Any slights of people, places, or organizations are unintentional.

First printing 1993

ISBN 0-9635554-4-8

LCCN 92-84076

Design, typesetting, and printing services provided by About Books, Inc., 425 Cedar Street, Buena Vista, CO 81211, 800-548-1876.

ATTENTION CORPORATIONS, COLLEGES, AND PRO-FESSIONAL ORGANIZATIONS: Quantity discounts are available on bulk purchases of this book for educational purposes or fund raising. Special books or book excerpts can also be created to fit specific needs. For information, please contact Sargasso Enterprises, 14 Wildwood Street, Winchester, MA 01890 or call 617-729-9037.

Dedicated to
Lauren Marie Belyea,
our friend.

Acknowledgments

I gratefully acknowledge the support, the expertise and the contributions of David, Matthew, and Catherine Krumme. They lived the book with me.

I further acknowledge the special efforts of David Krumme, Judie Muggia, Dr. Albert Muggia, Lori Lerman, and Ralene Walls who proofread the manuscript, offered suggestions and encouraged the effort.

I am grateful that the medical staff at the Massachusetts General Hospital Pediatric Oncology/Hematology Clinic were helpful and encouraging in this endeavor. They gave us hope and we thank them for our daughter.

I thank our friends and family for helping us, both then and now.

Cynthia A. Krumme

Contents

Foreword

Try to imagine that you are a healthy 4-year-old. You feel a little tired trying to keep up with your 6-year-old brother, and you get a few black-and-blues on your legs. You are given a blood test, and then you are taken into a big hospital for a needle in the back that is painful and frightening. Everybody is serious, and they tell you that you have a blood disease called leukemia. You need more shots and you start taking pills every day. Some days you feel worse than ever, and one day your hair starts to fall out. You look forward to the time when you are 7 and can stop taking pills and getting shots. Then when that time comes you learn that you can't stop. Instead you have to continue for another 3 years, and there are even more shots and worse side effects. Discouraging, yes. Disappointing, yes. Difficult to understand, yes. But does it slow you down, or get you down, or diminish your love of life? Not one bit.

This is the story of a remarkable little girl whom I first met during those difficult first days. Now she is 16 and as indomitable as ever. From her diaries, her parents' journals, her brother's essays, family letters, and the medical record, come the details of her story that are touching, frightening, maddening, ennobling, and above all, inspiring. She can teach all of us what a joyful thing life is. She can teach us how we can all respond to adversity, and how we can find the silver lining in every cloud. She can teach us how to approach life. Perhaps the "Clinic Rules" that she created, and are still on display at the clinic, can be paraphrased as rules to live by. They are worth examining in more detail:

1. *Must have a good sense of humor.* In the presence of hardship and adversity, your attitude may be your most important asset.

2. *Must always do a good LP and bone marrow.* This goes beyond mere technology, and reminds us that we should be competent in what we do because other people depend on us.

3. *Must always remember the toy box.* We must remember to remind those whom we love that we do love them even though from time to time we hurt them.

4. *Must tell the truth.* Concealing the truth makes a bad situation worse.

5. *Must like people.* It is others who will help us when it is our turn to face adversity.

6. *Must like junk food.* We must take time to enjoy the pleasant things in life.

7. *Must know a lot about chemotherapy.* We must know what we are talking about.

8. *Must not mind the sight of blood.* The unpleasant things in life must be faced whether we like it or not.

9. *Must like bald heads.* Ugliness is only in the eye of the beholder.

10. *Must never be grumpy.* Life is short and full of problems—a bad attitude only adds needlessly to the problems.

This is also the story of loving and determined parents who never gave up, who always looked ahead and who faced everything together. It is a tribute to intelligence, to devotion, to hard work, and above all to optimism. It is a story of the triumph of human will over adversity. It is a story that will inspire everyone who reads it, and will give courage to us all as we face the trials that we will inevitably face.

John Truman, M.D.

1

Relapse

As a family, we couldn't have felt happier than we did that day in November 1983 when seven-year-old Catherine finished her treatment for acute lymphocytic leukemia (ALL). I took her for the final tests that would satisfy the doctors that they were on solid ground in ending her chemotherapy and sending us off to be followed for four years of "social visits" to the clinic. Three years of business visits to the Pediatric Hematology/Oncology clinic had made us feel at home there. We knew many of the patients and had seen many old friends come and go: some ending treatment as we were about to do, others losing their long painful battles with cancer. We were comfortable with them all in a way that helped hold us all together. The bonds were strong.

The final spinal tap and bone marrow aspiration were dreaded by Catherine. Unfortunately the experience was unusually painful. Catherine described the spinal tap as causing her to feel as if she lost her mind. She finally asked Dr. Truman to stop: *Let me get my act together*. A measure of their mutual respect was that he did and she did. The bone marrow procedure went quite well. The tests were completed and congratulations were extended to and from our clinic friends; then we headed home to Winchester to meet David and to pick up nine-year-old Matthew from our friends' home where over the years he had spent so many days waiting for Catherine to come home from the clinic. On this special day, Judy and Paul broke out the champagne to celebrate the victory we had all fought so hard to achieve. After a joyful visit, our family took off for dinner at our favorite Chinese restaurant. At home that evening we all agreed it was wonderful to have no more pills, shots, IVs, or tests to go through, and none of the side effects of the chemotherapy. We talked about events that had happened and how we all felt now that the experience was mostly over. Both Catherine and Matthew fell into bed exhausted that evening, while David and I sat up and marveled at how much time had passed and what a mixture of joy and sadness our experience with cancer had been. We both felt badly that he had not been at the clinic that afternoon, both to help Catherine and to share in the excitement.

The next day we all enjoyed the pleasure of not beginning the day with a smorgasbord of medication. We also remembered that it was the third anniversary of the death of Danny, a small friend we knew from our first weeks at the clinic. The children set off for school, full of enthusiasm, planning to tell all their friends about the "family" achievement of the day before. David and I called our parents in Oklahoma and Louisiana and my sister in California to share the good news. Then they all got on the phone and relayed the good news to our widely dispersed families. That day, while making Catherine's bed, I found a note under her pillow. *I am glad I didn't die from leukemia.* That little note on lavender flowered paper in her childish handwriting tore the tears from me that had been just below the surface for days. We were so relieved, and clearly Catherine was too. The relief was very short lived.

The risk of relapse with leukemia diminishes with time. Seven years cancer-free is the benchmark associated with cure. In the case of ALL, the survival rate is continually improving, and at the time of Catherine's diagnosis, well over 50% of the children with Catherine's presentation of the disease survived. At the time of the last spinal and bone marrow, Dr. Truman told us her risk of relapse was about 10%.

At five p.m. Dr. Truman called the house. I was teaching a video production class and David was home from his Tufts University office and took the call. Dr. Truman said that the pathology lab had found 352 leukemia cells per milliliter of spinal fluid in the sample taken from Catherine on November 30. A relatively small amount, but enough to indicate a relapse. No cells were found in the bone marrow sample and the verdict was a central nervous system relapse. Dr. Truman expressed the hope that there had been a laboratory mistake and asked us to bring Catherine in early the next morning so they could repeat the tests. David asked him how often mistakes happened and he said, *very rarely.* He suggested that we begin to explain to the children what had happened and that we begin the process of adjusting to the diagnosis. After three years of adjusting, David knew some of what that meant. He asked Dr. Truman what the chances of recovery were for Catherine, given the type of relapse and her medical history. He told David that no more than one out of three children have a chance for complete control over this type of relapse. (The statistics commonly used at the time were 15 to 20%.) He briefly commented that the treatment would be brutal as the strongest measures were needed to bring a lasting remission.

When I returned home 30 minutes later, David's voice drifted down the stairs. His voice sounded urgent and strained. *Come up to your office now.* Tired from the day's work, I trudged up to my third floor office where a white faced husband and father had to tell a stricken wife and mother that her child had probably had a relapse of cancer. I remember clearly the unreal feeling of being in a nightmare and not believing what I was hearing. Even now it sometimes seems inconceivable that Catherine could have had cancer, let alone a relapse of the disease. David and I faced each other for a few minutes before I could ask any questions and before he could tell everything he had heard during that brief phone call. Time stopped for us briefly as we gave in to fear and grief, but just as has happened so many times before and since, the moment was over when we heard a little voice calling from downstairs, *Mommy, Daddy, where are you? What's for dinner?* In that moment, David and I agreed that the children should be told the situation and that we should join together to strengthen each other. We agreed to maintain hope and to offer it to both children. We knew we must begin again and that the strength we all had would be put to a severe test.

Downstairs in our warm kitchen, I took Catherine on my lap and told her about Dr. Truman's call. She sobbed, not fully realizing the impact of the diagnosis, but realizing that it meant at least three more years of chemotherapy and, beginning the next morning, more spinal taps, bone marrows, needles, and medicine. There was sorrow in her voice and pain in her eyes when she told us, *I'll be ten years old before it's over!* Our unspoken understanding was that what she feared was in fact the best possible scenario, one that was not the most probable. Matthew joined us and gravely listened to the situation. As he had done since both children were babies, he hugged his sister and tried to cheer her up. We could all only imagine what was coming, and each of us wrestled with our fears and deep feelings through that long night.

Innocence

That cold December night marked an end of a protective innocence which we had worn like a blanket: the innocence of total belief and surety of a cure with which we had covered ourselves for the three years following the original diagnosis in September 1980. We had all, family, friends, acquaintances, and insiders, pulled up that blanket whenever we needed it. It didn't prevent us from being realistic; it merely served to soften the impact. From my current vantage point, I know that for a family living with cancer in a child, there are several levels of acceptance, anger, coping, innocence, despair, growth, and hope that come and go during the process of living with cancer.

I'm moved to reconstruct the events we all refer to as Catherine's illness in the hope that the story will be helpful to other families and to Catherine and Matthew. This story belongs to them much more than to David and me, because they will be around long after we are not, and it is for them and all the other children that everyone has tried so hard. The story is full of ups and downs, successes and failures, gains and losses, sad and happy faces, little stories and big dreams, all mixed together and buoyed up with hope and expectation.

I began keeping a journal on September 26, 1980, on the express advice of a wonderful young woman I met during a hospital stay whose young son was dying. She walked into Catherine's room one afternoon and introduced herself and asked if there was anything she could do to help us. Her suggestion that I keep a journal was more help than she could imagine.

3

The Uneasy Summer

Leukemia surfaced in our household during the summer we contracted to paint the old house that we had moved into the previous summer. We began to see some subtle signs of illness in almost four-year-old Catherine in June, although it is only through hindsight that all those subtle signs become warnings. At the time, events were isolated, infrequent, and not troubling until late August. Matthew turned six in May of 1980 and for his birthday received a bicycle. Catherine, not wishing to be outdone, showed every sign of being ready to ride a bike too, so we bought one for her in June as an early birthday present. For weeks after, both children could be seen riding around the driveway with their training wheels barely touching the ground. Matthew got his training wheels off and one week later Catherine followed suit. We began to observe some small bruises and some not so small bruises on Catherine, which we attributed to the spills taken on the bike and to the general rough and tumble mode of play that the children enjoyed.

In early June, both children had their annual physical exams, complete with routine blood tests, and both were pronounced normal and healthy. We headed off for a long-planned trip to England in late June and stayed through July during which time we noticed that Catherine, who never took naps, began to take an occasional nap and was falling asleep early in the evening. We assumed that the vacation was tiring her out rather more than home did. Upon returning to the States, the house painter descended on our house and we took off for a week in Maine. Catherine was her old bouncy self throughout that week, but within days of returning home she was showing the same level of fatigue and once again developed some small bruises on her legs which were hard to account for. We surmised that she might be allergic to the dust and paint which was everywhere. A friend told me later that she and her doctor husband were disquieted by the bruises at that time. I wish they had spoken up, since it might have been helpful in getting her to the doctor sooner.

Throughout that long summer, I struggled with my own adjustments to being home after years of teaching, and to our new life in New England which was so different from our life in Berkeley. In short I felt restless and uneasy about a number of things, and Catherine's occasional bouts with fatigue just merged with the total picture. Like most parents of children with cancer, I sometimes think I would have been more suspicious or quicker to react to symptoms of leukemia if I had been less into myself that summer. What we all know is that sooner or later the symptoms of the disease cannot be missed, but I have not talked with any parents of children with cancer who did not question their own behavior in those few weeks before a diagnosis. Fortunately, early diagnosis is not as important with leukemia as it is with many other cancers.

As the beginning of September rolled around, my level of uneasiness about Catherine became overwhelming. I called for an appointment with our pediatrician at Harvard Community Health Plan. I described the symptoms and my vague concerns to the nurse, who suggested I wait three days until Dr. Keefer would be back from jury duty. Those three days dragged by. Several people commented on how pale Catherine appeared to be. Finally on a Thursday afternoon we piled into the car (I insisted that David come along), and off we went to see the doctor, convinced that she would offer some perfectly reasonable solution as to why Catherine was having these problems. We noticed that day that Catherine had developed some small red spots just under her eyes and was running a low grade fever. Neither David nor I ever suspected leukemia, although we had both known children with the disease from my school in California, and we knew well the terrifying story of an old friend's child who was diagnosed in 1965 and died in just two weeks.

Our little family took seats in a small office at HCHP in Cambridge and within 15 minutes we heard the word cancer whispered to us by Dr. Keefer. Catherine sat demurely on the big examination table, with Matthew standing beside her and David and me watching Dr. Keefer look Catherine over. She surveyed an ugly bruise on her left leg, asked several questions regarding Catherine's behavior, and then suggested that we get a blood test and return to her office. After that first blood test, an ordeal for a frightened four-year-old, we returned to the office. Dr. Keefer told us it would take some time for the test results to come back and that we should go home and wait for her call. She said she suspected cancer. The impact of those words and the feeling of that moment are still with us.

Beginnings

David and I looked at the doctor, and at each other, and at our beloved children, and I quietly resolved to live with what had happened in the best way I could. We took deep breaths, smiled at the children, thanked the doctor, and told her we would be expecting her call. Both children climbed into the car and began happily discussing how hungry they were. *Let's go to McDonald's for cheeseburgers!* Somehow we drove to the restaurant, ordered the food, and swallowed it. I barely remember anything except a vague feeling of eating cardboard. At home we explained to Catherine that we would be going to see another doctor in the morning and that everything was going to be all right. At 9 p.m., Dr. Keefer called to confirm a tentative diagnosis of leukemia. She confirmed our appointment for 11:00 the next morning at the Massachusetts General Hospital clinic of Dr. John Truman. She explained that Dr. Truman was in South America, but his associate Dr. John Curnutte was expecting us. She wished us well and answered my only question, *Do children survive this disease?* with a firm yes. She has since told us that Catherine was her first cancer diagnosis and that she was impressed with the hopeful spirit that we expressed. In our view there was no other way to look at the situation. At that point, hope was all we had.

We hardly slept that night. David cried and I comforted him. He poured out his grief all at once, while I doled mine out gradually over the years. We both railed against the gross unfairness of the situation. We had almost no information to go on, but we clung to the idea that children could be cured. We discovered as early in the process as that first night that each of us had very different adjustment requirements, but just being together was a good start. In the morning we tried to be cheerful. We made arrangements for Matthew after school and tried to listen enthusiastically to his excitement about his first full day of first grade. After driving him to school, getting one last hug and reassuring him that we would all be fine, I returned home. I found David setting up his drums in the living room for Catherine to play, an activity that she had never been allowed before as she was not old enough to play with real instruments. She was thrilled. As she banged on the drums trying to imitate her daddy, our eyes filled with tears at the thought that this might be her last chance.

Eager to get on with it, we headed in to the clinic at the Mass. General where we were shown to the waiting room by the young, very blond receptionist named Cindy. She reassured us, made Catherine smile, and told us to relax and that the doctors would be along soon. Within a few minutes of meeting Dr. Curnutte and Monica, the clinic nurse, we had learned that medicine had advanced dramatically in the treatment of childhood leukemia, that there are many forms of childhood leukemia, that the initial presentation of the disease varies drastically, and that they both thought that Catherine was adorable. We liked them immediately.

Friday, September 12, 1980 was the first day of Catherine's exposure to the sometimes painful, often frightening, frequently boring, and always eventful world of the cancer clinic. At barely four years of age she faced the abrupt end of her uncluttered childhood and the beginning of an artificially imposed maturity full of stressful demands.

The battery of tests given Catherine included blood tests to monitor the impact of the disease on all blood components, a spinal tap, also called a lumbar puncture or LP, designed to check for leukemic cells in the spinal fluid, a bone marrow aspiration from the hip to count the leukemic cells in the site of blood production, and chest X-rays to detect any possible spread of cancer cells to the lymph nodes in the chest. The LP and the bone marrow tests, each consisting of the insertion of a long needle deep into tissue and bone to extract fluid and marrow, were extremely painful. All of the tests were used in determining the exact nature of the leukemia in order to design the most effective treatment program. Understanding the need for all of this, David and I stood with her, held her hand when possible, and tried to comfort her, console her, and explain why four adults needed to hold her down and stick needles into her arm, back, and hip. Her platelet count was so low that each stick bled profusely. Pressure bandages were necessary over the LP and bone marrow sites to stop the blood flow. Catherine was terribly frightened. I am still not sure how we got through that day, but by the end of it Catherine was bravely assisting in her treatment.

At some point during that long day I read a message on the clinic bulletin board that said:

> *How do I feel? Don't ask! . . . aside from nervousness, irritability, exhaustion, faintness, dizziness, tremor, cold sweats, depression, insomnia, muscle pains, mental confusion, internal trembling, numbness, indecisiveness, crying spells, unsocial, asocial and anti-social behavior . . . I feel fine . . . Thank you.*

People in cancer clinics behave as if the world were normal. They take coffee breaks, eat lunch, tell jokes, and laugh just as if the world were going to advance as always. We were amazed then, and are still amazed, at the resiliency of the human spirit. After the initial tests we were sent to eat lunch and await a consultation with the doctor. We located the hospital snack bar and ordered food. Catherine was hungry and I believe comforted by the normal act of eating lunch. While we sat there, the actress Lee Remick walked in and sat at our table. Her father was in the hospital and I remember thinking that she looked as bewildered as we felt. It was vaguely reassuring to know that famous people had real problems too, and that they chose the Mass. General for treatment when they could go anywhere.

At 4 p.m., David and I met in conference with Dr. Curnutte while Catherine crawled under the waiting room chairs and fell asleep, her little blue jean skirt with its pink and blue flowers tucked around her protectively. We looked at her with tears in our eyes and then got down to business.

Dr. Curnutte explained the types of leukemia to us, indicated that it would require further evaluation to determine the exact type that Catherine had, and said that the exact treatment would be determined by which kind of white blood cell was involved. He indicated that she would begin chemotherapy as an outpatient on Monday, September 15. Catherine had a fever of 100.4, a hematocrit of 16.7, a platelet count of 31,000, and a white cell count of 27,000. (Normal for a child of four is in the 35 range for the hematocrit, over 150,000 platelets, and between 4,000 and 10,000 white cells.) We discussed the possibility of blood transfusions and we were warned of the possibility of a hospital admission earlier than Monday if her fever went up. This was our introduction to the clinic philosophy which included living as normally as possible, staying out of the hospital whenever possible, and being active partners in the treatment process.

From the *MGH News* article by Linda Goodspeed, December 1991:

> *"It doesn't do much good to cure patients of leukemia only to have them scarred in other ways," Dr. Ferguson added. "By and large the children are able to carry on normal lives, and we encourage them to do so."*

We asked a few tentative questions: *How long will the medicine be given? When will the red spots on the skin (petechiae) go away? How much blood will she need?* We were told in clear terms as much information as we could hold. Nurse Monica looked after all of us in an efficient, affectionate way. It was she who first asked, *Has Catherine had the chicken pox?* This issue would haunt us for several years, although at the time it seemed unimportant. Dr. Curnutte gave us packages of prednisone, allopurinol, and Bactrim, the first in what would be an endless trail of pills to swallow, in this instance designed to prepare her body for the onslaught of chemotherapy, and he also gave us his most optimistic appraisal of the situation. He gave us the clinic's business card with its 24-hour phone number, and he carefully explained that we were her best first defense against problems such as low blood counts, other side effects of chemotherapy, and even the possibility of a relapse going unnoticed. If she had a fever over 101 degrees, complained strongly of pain in her bones or anywhere else, appeared sick, or if we were just concerned, we were to call the clinic. With our tired, hurt little girl in tow, we obediently headed home.

Cynthia Krumme

5

We Have to Tell Everyone

Even before we had a formally confirmed diagnosis we realized that we had to begin notifying family and friends. All our family members live in other parts of the country. Everyone's reaction was of shock and horror, and it was sometimes overwhelming to us, yet we desperately needed the love and support that followed. Our first call went to David's parents in Oklahoma. It was heart-breaking to have to tell them what had happened. They volunteered to come for a few days to take care of Matthew. They took the first plane out and arrived in time to pick up Matthew from his best friend's home after school, while we were in Boston at the clinic for the first time. Mimi and Grandad stayed for a week.

That first night our neighbors dropped in to tell us about their new table saw and walked away in stunned silence with our news. We called friends to make plans for Matthew for the next day and received from them the assurance that our dear son would always be welcome at their home any time, any day, for any reason. We have taken them up on that loving offer many times over the years and honor them greatly for helping us help Matthew have a normal life. Both these couples, among many others, have been stalwart, and both helped us notify other friends, thereby sparing us the stress of that job.

We called my brother in Louisiana and enlisted his aid in telling my parents, both of whom had been ill. In addition to making the first move with them, he called my sister in California. Later in the evening and many times over the next few days we spoke to them all. It was a significant problem not to have family members nearby, since it put us in the position of having to ask friends and acquaintances for aid that in many instances would come automatically from family. We found over the years that some people cope well with this type of problem and some do not, and we found this to be true of family members, friends, and people we came across in day to day living.

We have also come to see that it is difficult to be far away and fully appreciate what is going on. This applies equally to maintaining hope, sharing pain, and appreciating the imposed lifestyle of the patient and family. We found it helpful to keep people regularly informed of the progress, which we did with frequent phone calls, letters, and cards. I think it helped us all.

Our friends in our small town rallied, sending hopeful words, food, offers of help, and surprises for Catherine. Support came in letters from friends in California. Calls came with offers of grocery shopping, babysitting, errand running, advice about treatment centers, and general words of encouragement and affection. The initial support was heartfelt, helpful, and overwhelming. We were deluged with calls of condolence and offers of help. We felt conspicuous and singled out, whereas we were accustomed to being inconspicuous. It was hard to respond to so many offers of help and so many questions. We did not know what to say. Nothing seemed enough. Though it was terribly difficult to explain again and again what had happened, I believe it was useful and necessary in helping us to accept the reality of the situation and to begin to get down to business. While it was sometimes difficult to accept the outpouring of help, it would have been devastating to have had no offers of help. While heart-breaking to tell what happened, it would have been horrible to have no one to listen. Those who have lived through similar situations will understand. Thank you is not enough.

Notes and messages arrived daily and they brought affection and words of support which were very helpful.

We are all sorry to hear you are not feeling well. Please get well soon. Your friends can't wait till you are A-OK again.

Please don't hesitate to call if you would like some instant food, drink, available ears etc. etc.

I've heard through the "jungle telegraph" of your little girl's illness. I was really sorry to hear it. I've been through times like that myself and I really do know what you're going through. I remember thinking that no matter what happened I would never be really happy again. Well, I was wrong. I have been and I am. Marge said she saw you the other day and that you looked and sounded really good. I'm so glad. And the prognosis I understand is very positive. I'm glad for you. I send you my love, my energy and some of the faith I found—faith that you will be happy again. That must be faith in the human spirit I guess. Or faith in the strength we find in ourselves and that we get from those who love us. Have faith!

Since I'm thinking of you and your little girl constantly, I might as well tell you so and hope it adds to the moral support flowing in from all your friends and from those who care.

Your letter arrived today and ever since you have all been in my thoughts. My initial response was tearful grief. I feel helpless so far from you. I wish I was there to give daily support—to help you cry and to help you laugh. To cheer Catherine on for every good day she has and to reassure and comfort her for each not so good day. Call anytime you need to talk. I love you all and send a hug as wide as the sky.
Love

Talking about leukemia and understanding our reactions and the reactions of others has been a primary focus of our energies over the years. As time passed and emotions changed and fatigue set in and the long haul became the reality, we experienced many difficult moments with our own feelings and with the feelings and actions of others. We are all complex people; there is no "right way" to experience cancer, but we have come to understand and to accept most of what has happened. We are buoyed up with the long term friendly help, with no strings attached, that was given by a few special families. They have little if any awareness of how special their gestures have been, but the very fact that sometimes they just said, *Don't worry, we'll do that,* without ever being asked or asking for any explanations was a gift beyond measure.

The Hospital Admission

By Saturday noon all the immediate calls had been made and both children had been told the name of the illness and that we would have to work very hard together to help Catherine get well. They were stoic and so were we. Catherine and I spent the first of many hours practicing taking pills—not so easy for a four-year-old. In the end she took her assorted pills more or less ground up in applesauce and agreed to try to swallow the next ones. Much to her delight and ours she learned to take pills in a matter of three or four days. Already Catherine showed every sign of taking charge of her own illness.

From Matt's college essay, Fall 1991:

> *I can remember the first time I watched Catherine taking pills, just after her diagnosis. A dozen pills lay on the table, arranged by their color and size. She courageously swallowed all the pills, and I remarked that I was bigger than she was but that I couldn't even swallow one pill.*

My parents called to offer encouragement and to suggest that I purchase her a new nightgown and robe from them. I went out and did so, but can scarcely remember the trip. David's parents were loving, supportive, and helpful, and I am convinced that their presence in our midst helped us get through those first bleak days.

At 11:00 Saturday night, Catherine's temperature hit 102, and, as instructed, we headed in to the Mass. General. We wrapped Catherine in her new pink wooly robe, gathered up her favorite bear Freddy, and carried her out of the comfort and security of her house to the terror of the hospital. During that drive, I was alone with

David and the sleeping child, and the full impact began to sink in. I was afraid.

Catherine was admitted to the hospital through the emergency room. It was the first of several admissions due to fever of indeterminate origin. We were up all night getting X-rays, blood tests, blood transfusions, and speaking to doctor after doctor. The entire experience was a nightmare. The insertion of a large IV needle was necessary, of course, and Catherine was frightened. The doctor, whose initial manner was pleasant and friendly, had difficulty with the IV. Catherine screamed hysterically. The doctor became agitated, missed the IV again, and finally made David and me leave the room. He called in others to hold her down, and he put in the IV while she screamed like a trapped animal. Many painful and frightening things have been necessary since that first IV, but we have never since accepted being told to leave as we did that night. There was no life threatening situation going on, only a tired and sick child expressing her fear. Everyone in that room learned from that experience. The fear was with her for several weeks, and although she spoke maturely of understanding the need for the IV, by morning she was asking her father to find her yellow baby blanket and to bring it soon. From that time on we have acted as advocates for her; many times it has been necessary to speak up for her rights. The yellow blanket stayed with her for years, always brought out when a little additional edge was needed.

Catherine's hematocrit was only 14 and she was given two blood transfusions and admitted to the Intensive Care Unit. It was four in the morning before she was settled in a bed, hooked up to every monitoring device available, and allowed to sleep. David and I were interviewed by a young doctor who took an entire medical history, which included family histories of cancer and other chronic diseases, Catherine's birth history, details of her bout at age two months with viral spinal meningitis, and a complete review of the leukemia history. We found this a little tedious at 3:00 a.m. but we complied. We were told that Dr. Truman would return to Boston on Monday and that he would tell us the cell type of Catherine's leukemia and would outline the treatment which would begin Monday night, assuming her fever went down and her red blood count went up. That particular doctor's easy manner relaxed us. I remember that we even laughed with him over some small thing. David went home to be with Matthew and I sat up all night in a rocking chair. Through the connecting door, I watched silently as the young car accident victim in the next room labored to stay alive and I hoped for the life of our darling girl. Many times since that long night we have discussed the difficulties of the hospital routine where everything goes on from life-and-death struggles to mundane house cleaning chores, with little regard to day or night. It is an unreal world all its own. From that time on, we knew that the hospital, despite being a wonderful place with caring skilled staff people, was to be avoided if at all possible.

On Sunday Catherine was feeling much better. After the two units of blood, her red cell count was 21, and the doctor indicated we were to be transferred to the children's ward on Monday whenever they could get a bed. So began a routine that would govern our lives for nearly seven years. David and I took turns staying with our children, sleeping in the hospital and taking care of home business. For us this sharing of responsibility was important and I believe that it was a major factor in keeping the family normal and in minimizing the stress that we all experienced.

Despite difficulties in obtaining a bed, Catherine was moved to the children's ward on Burnham 5 at midday on Monday. Since no actual room was available, her bed was placed in the playroom, and it was there at about five in the afternoon that we met John Truman and learned the full impact of the diagnosis. Dr. Truman, a tall, thin dignified man in his early forties, was delightful, soft spoken, and calm. He charmed us from the beginning, and our faith in him was established from that first meeting. Catherine was sleeping soundly in the rolling hospital bed with all of us standing around her while he confirmed the diagnosis of acute lymphocytic leukemia, null cell type. We were assured that this was the most common childhood leukemia and the statistics were most favorable for its successful treatment. At that time, September 1980, the cure rate for null cell ALL was expected to be around 65%, with a 35% failure rate. He told us that 5% of the failed cases never responded to treatment. I remember thinking that anything less than a 100% cure rate was not good enough. During this discussion, he made it clear to us that a remission is much easier to achieve than a cure, but that both were doable.

Dr. Truman described the induction chemotherapy which would begin immediately with the goal of remission within 30 days, and he mentioned the sanctuary phase of treatment which usually included full cranial radiation. He mentioned that there were some long-term side-effects of cranial radiation. I felt as if a truck had run over me. I asked Dr. Truman whether there were any other options. He said he had heard that Catherine was very bright and he was looking forward to speaking with her and that he would discuss options with us later. I remember very well how odd it felt to be holding such a discussion in a playroom.

From Catherine's medical records, September 15, 1980:

> *Decision whether or not to randomize to regimen 1 or 2 can wait until maintenance phase is reached. Alternative to cranial radiation discussed in broad terms, as parents concerned about future CNS effects of RT and ITMTX. This could be intermediate-dose MTX per CALGB protocol #7911. J. Truman.* (We learned that treatment protocols were organized as nationwide scientific experiments; thus CALGB #7911 would be one of the regimens controlled by Cancer and Leukemia Group B.)

Catherine woke up and was her cheerful self. She responded to Dr. Truman's questions, let him examine her, and asked him when she would get some food and a room. She liked him and he liked her. Within a few minutes of his leaving, a room was found for Catherine, and within the hour she had received her first chemotherapy consisting of methotrexate, asparaginase, and vincristine by IV and prednisone and allopurinol by mouth. Other than fatigue and some irritability, the only other effects were a mild headache and a short bout of vomiting two days later. We learned that the side effects of chemotherapy can vary drastically from person to person and from dose to dose. Since that first chemotherapy, we tried to assume that she would feel fine most of the time. We believe that this upbeat attitude helped minimize the apprehension that is normal when facing chemo and may well have helped her to cope better. During that first hospital stay we all noticed the effects of being in the hospital more than the effects of chemo. We were accepted into a four bed room and Catherine was treated well by everyone. David and I took turns sleeping in a chair by her bed, neither of us wishing to leave her there alone at her age. During that week we met Sheryl and her eighteen-month-old son Danny who was being treated for acute mylogenous leukemia.

After six days in the hospital, Catherine was released with no fever on Thursday, Sept. 18. The bright spot of that week was going home.

From Catherine's medical records, September 17, 1980:

Gratifying decrease in WBC and spleen size. Home tomorrow. J. Truman.

In late 1981 at age 5, Catherine dictated this story about her illness.

My Leukemia

I first got leukemia when I was four years old. We went to Maine and I had my fourth birthday there. I took a lot of naps there even though I had already given them up. When we came home I started riding my two wheeled bike and I got a lot of bruises when I was riding my bike. My mom thought that they were ordinary bruises. We called up the Harvard Health Plan and they said to come and see them. Then my mom noticed that I had a little fever too. I didn't even feel sick. My doctor said to go to the hospital to see some special doctors. The HCHP doctor told my mom and dad that I might have leukemia. They told us to go home and wait until tomorrow to see the special doctors. That night we had cheeseburgers to eat. My brother and I love cheeseburgers! We went home to bed and the next morning we went to the Mass General. First I went to get a blood test. I had a bone marrow after that. Then we went to eat lunch in the cafeteria. Mom and Dad shared a coke and I had another cheeseburger and a coke to drink and some yogurt. Then we went back upstairs and I had some X-rays. We had a long time to wait but we got to talk to Dr. Curnutte, Monica and Cindy. I was so tired that I went to sleep on the floor. Mommy and Daddy had a meeting with the doctors. Mom and Dad carried me home and we found my grandparents at home waiting to help out. I liked it that they came. They came to baby-sit my brother Matthew if I had to go to the hospital and stay there for a while. That night my parents told me that I had leukemia. I wanted to know if they would take care of me. They said they would and that the doctors would help us all. They said I would be getting medicine called chemotherapy. We started right out with learning to take some pills that the doctor said I needed before we could start the chemotherapy on Monday. I wasn't very good at taking pills because the pill was sticky because I left it in my mouth for a long time. It wasn't very long before I got over that.

The next night I got a high fever. We called the hospital and they told us what to do. They said that we should come to the emergency room at the hospital and we did. My mom had bought me a pretty pink robe and she put it on me to go to the hospital. I was very scared going to the emergency room and having the IV. It was very late at night and I was very sleepy. I was so scared by the IV that I cried and the doctor said that if I did not stop crying that my mom and dad would be sent out of the room. I didn't stop crying and the doctor sent my mom and dad out of the room. I didn't like it but he put in the IV anyway. It made me feel sad and my mom and dad too. Ever since then my mom and dad stay in the room, help me, and stay close by me. I think that it is better to have your parents with you. Since I was feeling sick I had to stay several nights in the hospital. I went to Burnham 5. I liked to play in the playroom there. I got my first chemotherapy there. I know that I get chemotherapy so that I will get better. Monica and Dr. Truman said that they would help me get better. I believe them. Mom and Dad

Cynthia Krumme

stayed with me in the hospital. They take turns spending the night with me and with my brother Matthew. After a while I got to go home and I had a bunch of pills to take and Mommy said that I had to go back to get IVs.

My first day home I went straight to nursery school. I was feeling better. My grandmother Mimi and my grandfather went home after I came home from the hospital. In the beginning I was pretty scared of the IVs. They hurt me. After a while I learned to have IVs without crying so much. Here is my secret. I sit quietly and don't get hysterical and do some deep breathing out and in and think happy thoughts and look at my mother's face. We breathe together, but I can do it by myself. The IV still hurts but it is not so bad and soon it is over.

Nursery School and Normal Life

Catherine went straight to her nursery school classroom from the hospital that Thursday. In her second year at the school, she loved the teachers and loved being with her friends. We had spoken to the director, made an attempt to explain the situation, and asked for notification in the event of chicken pox cases or exposures at the school. The parents had been informed of the situation by the school newsletter which we found posted on the door as we entered. It shocked me to see Catherine's name and the word leukemia in the same sentence. One of the continuing problems facing our family and other families was the extreme public nature of the life that we had to lead in order to help Catherine experience a normal, active childhood.

GOOD NEWS! Catherine Krumme's doctors report that she has the mildest of the several forms of leukemia. The prognosis is good and treatment will also be milder than some forms of treatment. She could be back at school quite soon although treatment will continue on an outpatient basis.

You have all been so caring in your response to Catherine and Cindy and Dave and Matthew—I thought you would want to share this happy news.

Leukemia patients cannot get chicken pox—the result could be fatal. Please let us know if your child has been exposed or if a sibling has chicken pox—then Catherine will not come to school—will not risk exposure.

P.S. Please don't call the Krummes for a while—life is a bit hectic. We have just learned that blood donations in Catherine's behalf would be welcome anytime at Mass General—Give Catherine's name. There will also be a Bloodmobile on Sept. 27—details later.

This awkward first foray back into the "real world" marked the beginning of another phase of adjustment for us. We realized that our lives were now in the public domain more than they had ever been. We encountered supportive behavior from many people and critical behavior from others. We have observed over the years that some people find the ability to help in every instance and others criticize even the smallest perceived mistake.

Most people were happy to see us at the school, but not all were. The strongest reaction was *What are you doing here? I could never bring my child from the hospital to school!* I admit to being totally amazed to this day that anyone would question our decisions at that point. It is clear to me that such reactions are fairly normal and well within the range of strange things that happen to families with chronically or critically ill children. The presence of such children places an added emotional burden on people, and people react in a variety of ways.

On that first day back, Catherine sat down at her little table and absorbed the events around her. She drew a picture of her family together, surrounding her, smiling and leaning in toward her protectively. Her drawing gave great hope to David and me. If she could feel as loved and protected as the picture indicated after the week she had experienced, then surely she could carry on her battle successfully. She had a wonderful afternoon at school.

Despite our best efforts to keep Catherine's life normal, in January we took her out of the private, parent-cooperative nursery school. Chicken pox exposures began and some parents began to feel uneasy about the risks and apparently unable to allow us, as Catherine's parents, in connection with her doctors, to determine when the exposure was dangerous to her. The nature of cancer treatment is that the patient and family have little control over anything. Life seems totally out of control in fact. Whether

Catherine went to school on a given day was one thing we felt should be within our control. We could not deal with the idea that the school would tell us whether Catherine could come on any given day. We were offended by the suggestion that Catherine would be prevented from attending school because the other parents would feel guilty if Catherine were to be exposed to the chicken pox by one of their children. This situation could only have arisen in a private school; in a public school, she would have a legal right to attend. The school administration felt uneasy, and was especially responsive to the parents' concerns because of the democratic nature of the school's governance. Unfortunately communication broke down at a time when we were unable to devote the energy required to reach an understanding. We felt that we already had enough battles to wage, and so we withdrew from the school even though Catherine loved it there. This episode was heartbreaking for us and hurtful to many others who seemed not to understand our attempts to explain and still don't. Regretfully for everyone, no intervention occurred to try to work things out. This remains a sad chapter for us.

From the Journal, January 6, 1981:

Apparently people cannot let us take the responsibility for deciding when to take the risk of chicken pox exposure or not, as they feel they would be overcome with guilty feelings if their child exposed Catherine to chicken pox and she got very sick or worse. How can this be happening?

Uncertainty

My journals say a lot about those turbulent first few weeks of Catherine's treatment. At the time of her second chemotherapy treatment on Monday the 22nd, she still had very few platelets, which required extra caution to prevent bruising, but her hematocrit was up and her white count was down. The initial dose of chemo was powerful and its impact on the leukemic cells was profound.

The IV for Monday's chemo was very difficult and required four attempts before a vein could be secured. As with all young children, her veins were small and the skill required to find them was immense. We have marveled over the years at the small number of poor IV sticks. Most of the perfect sticks have been administered by nurses.

At the clinic it was noted that Catherine had an infected cut on her elbow, not surprising considering her low white count. However, as a new clinic mother, nervous and fearful like all new parents in the clinic, I interpreted the staff concern over the cut as a criticism of my diligence and vowed to be scrupulously cautious in the future. To put this reaction in perspective, the clinic for new families can be a harrowing experience. "Old timers" are accustomed to being in a situation where children are sick, crying, recovering, laughing, screaming, and in some instances dying. The clinic was, and still is occasionally, a hard experience. There is pain of all kinds, mixed with the tremendous sense of hope, the excellent medical treatment, and the occasional hilarious events that occur there. On day 9 of our new life it still hadn't really sunk in how much a part of our lives this clinic would be.

From Catherine's medical records, September 26, 1980:

Explained that hospitalization changes children for a while. Catherine also blaming mother for their trips to clinic. Mom and Catherine talk over all procedures. Catherine clinging to Mom. Monica Corrigan, RN.

David went to work and Matthew trudged the mile to his school and attended first grade. For him, the sacrifices began early and have been made lovingly ever since. From the homemade get well cards sent to the hospital, to the hugs for his sister each day as he left for school, he shouldered his share of the family responsibility well. Siblings are included from the start in our clinic and an open invitation was extended to Matthew to join us there. In an attempt to keep his life as normal as possible, we decided that school would come first. His first grade teacher reported to us that he was doing well, and Judy and Paul, our good friends who watched over him, reported that he was hanging in there just like the rest of us. These reports lifted our spirits.

On day 13 we went to the clinic for a check up and blood test and were introduced to a 23-year-old man who had leukemia 13 years before and was cured. He looked wonderful! I decided to seek out success stories and read everything I could get my hands on regarding treatment and the experiences of others.

From the Journal, September 26, 1980:

The clinic is filled with hope and despair. I am slow to accept and deal with all that has happened. I feel like a shell going through the motions of reassuring everyone while I am so unsure myself. I am envious of what seems to be David's calm acceptance. I am tired of talking about leukemia, yet if anyone asks I just pour out detail after detail.

By this time Catherine was showing the physical effects of prednisone more than any of the other medicines. A steroid that enhances the anti-cancer effect of vincristine, prednisone increased her appetite, caused body swelling, and contributed to mood swings. She could sit down at the table and eat nonstop until we made her leave the food alone. It was very frustrating for her and for us. In the early days she cried for food. We tried to exercise caution about what she ate but frequently found ourselves giving her more than we felt was appropriate. We had to unlearn the pre-leukemia ways and learn the new ways. Prednisone was unpleasant for Catherine throughout her treatment. She hated the taste and the side effects. In the first four weeks of prednisone, Catherine gained five pounds on her 40 pound body.

From Catherine's notes dictated at age 6:

I was taking prednisone a lot in the beginning and it made me chubby. I was hungry all the time. Every time I get prednisone now, it still makes me hungry.

From Catherine's story after nearly three years of treatment, September 1983:

I took a lot of prednisone. It made me a bit chubby which I don't like. It causes lots of problems while it is helping me. A big problem, which not many people know about, is it makes my underwear too tight because I get chubby and they are small around the waist. I have two wardrobes; one for prednisone and one for regular times. Even though I get chubby it does go away after a while. I'm happy when it does.

Prednisone was a problem for every family we met. Chad Green, a child removed from conventional leukemia treatment by his young parents and taken to Mexico for laetrile and enzyme enemas, was from our clinic. His parents reported that the drugs given him at the clinic, particularly prednisone, were destroying his personality and causing him too much pain. They described uncontrolled behavior and voracious appetites. Chad died. With conventional treatment, he might have lived. This case was prominently discussed by the television news and major newspapers throughout the country.

On the 16th day, when I told Catherine it was a clinic day, her apprehension showed. She startled noticeably and her cheeks turned scarlet and stayed that way all the way into the clinic. This became a common response to going in for treatment, even though she would remain agreeable and even cheerful. At the clinic she was uneventfully given vincristine by IV, and Dr. Truman outlined the second (sanctuary) stage of treatment. We were given the alternative treatment option of intermediate-dose methotrexate: methotrexate administered in high doses intravenously so that the blood-brain barrier would be overcome and that leukemic cells in the brain and spinal fluid would be killed, instead of the more standard treatment of radiation therapy in which radiation is directly applied to the brain to kill the leukemic cells. Both treatment options have risks and neither is perfect. At the time we were told that the risks of radiation on a four-year-old included some minor but permanent brain damage in some of the cases. The main risk of the methotrexate option was that it would be less effective against the leukemia. I felt overwhelmed again by the dismal choices. Since opting for neither was not a choice, we elected the chemotherapy option. At home that night Catherine had a nose bleed that took nearly an hour to stop. We had never seen a nose that bled so much or for so long. We were all frightened by the severity of the bleed. A call to the clinic was reassuring.

From the medical records, October 14, 1980:

> *Parents have carefully weighed pros and cons of intermediate-dose methotrexate vrs. cranial radiation and accepted CNS treatment CALGB # 7911. J. Truman.*

Catherine began to ask every day if it was a clinic day. She often had an expression of hurt on her face, she carried her teddy bear and her blanket around with her at home, and she crawled into bed frequently to sleep. She still cried and begged us to stop when the IVs were put in, but she held still as if she knew that it would happen anyway and the one thing she could control was her own reaction. She was growing older by the minute, her childhood changing along with her acceptance of her illness.

As the days went by we resumed normal social activities, put in a new fence, reveled in each other's company, and worried about some mundane things for a change. At the one month mark David commented that we only had 35 months to go. We felt good about the progress! An acquaintance with a chronically ill child herself organized a clinic day food service for us. It was very kind and very helpful.

In an attempt to get a better picture of leukemia in general and Catherine's prospects in specific, we searched every resource available to us. We went to libraries and book stores, scoured the clinic reference books, and asked questions. We read every book written about families and leukemia. I worried over the emotional well being of my children. *Would they develop normally? Were we spending enough time with them? Was Matthew being treated fairly? Would Catherine remember only pain? Could we live a normal life with cancer in the family?* The answers just evolved over time.

From the Journal, October 6, 1980:

A friend's father just died of cancer. I am sure that the spectre of his cancer was much more of a burden for her than we knew. I am just beginning to realize how difficult living with a long term illness will be. I have made some tentative resolves that I hope will help ease the stress for me. When casual acquaintances ask how Catherine is doing, I'm going to say just fine. I will elaborate only if they press me. This might help lift the burden of continually thinking about the illness. Catherine's cancer is much more difficult and horrible to live with than I am able to tell anyone else.

Remission

The journal I kept was a great comfort to me especially on clinic days. Early in Catherine's treatment, the days are marked clearly and are highlighted by long rambling essays which record my questions, fears, confusions and expectations. I was prolific on clinic days.

After four weeks of induction chemotherapy including six days in the hospital, weekly trips for checkups, and the daily round of pill taking, the day to test the hoped-for and expected remission was at hand. We were all filled with dread, both of the spinal and bone marrow tests and of the frightening possibility that we were not successful. Catherine asked directly if she was going to have the tests that day and we told her what to expect.

From the Journal, October 14, 1980:

> *I really don't know any way to handle this whole business properly. Does anyone? My instincts must be the guide. I've decided to try to erase the self pity as much as possible from all of us. Our life now is little different really. We go about our business and work the clinic into our lives.*

The remission visit began with a routine blood test and ended with a bone marrow aspiration and spinal tap. The results were excellent and Dr. Truman gleefully pronounced her bone marrow to be clear. His enthusiasm was electrifying and we all felt charged with optimism.

Dr. Elizabeth Robbins joined us that day for the first time. Her quiet reassurance during the spinal tap was helpful in calming Catherine's fears. Monica held our girl as we stood next to her head and held her hands. It remains a sharp hurt in my heart to recall the trauma of the treatment for our child at those times. We had a lengthy discussion of what would be happening next, and Dr. Truman indicated that if her long blond hair had not fallen out by now, it might not come out. Fear of losing her hair was very real to her and the possibility that she might not lose it made her very happy.

From Catherine's dictation age 6:

I had been getting vincristine for a while, my mom says four weeks, and it was time to test to see if I was better. We went to get a bone marrow test and it hurt, but my parents hugged me all through it and then it was over. Dr. Truman took the marrow to the microscope and looked at it and after a while he looked and cried out "Perfect." I figured it would be all right, but my mom and dad were very happy.

David was not able to go to the clinic for every visit, but he attempted to go whenever possible and always when major tests were scheduled. He was a well-known father at the clinic where fathers were seen less frequently than mothers. In those early days I felt that he had recovered from the shock of the diagnosis better than I, and often I thought I needed to get over it. That evening he told me that he felt it difficult to spend a day at the clinic, and that the day had given him new sympathy for the uneasiness that I had been expressing. Over the years we have been able for the most part to openly express our fears and feelings to each other. It has sometimes been difficult to express our fear, anxiety, or resentment when these emotions surfaced, but we have worked at it. I believe that this has helped our family handle all the experiences we have been through. That evening we joined Judy and Paul for dinner, and Catherine and David went with her friend Mark and Paul to "special friends" night at their nursery school while Matthew and Jeff played with "Transformers." It was a wonderful contrast to the clinic.

From the Journal, October 15, 1980:

Watching all the children at the clinic is very hard. Some of them are dying. Some of the teenagers are very weak and one young man breaks my heart. Yesterday his skin was green, but he jokes and talks with Dr. Truman, who lets him smoke without a word of reproach. We have entered the world of survivors, victims, and pain, and Catherine is our shining star.

From a letter to Dr. Keefer, HCHP, from Dr. Truman, October 16, 1980:

It's a great pleasure to report that Catherine Krumme's bone marrow is back to normal and she has entered complete remission. She now enters the cranio-spinal phase and the family has opted for intravenous methotrexate instead of cranial radiation. This is still in the quasi-experimental phase, although we have been using it on selected patients since 1976. It involves three 24-hour admissions for a moderately high dose of IV methotrexate followed the next day by citrovorum factor rescue. When this is finished, she begins the maintenance phase which requires only one visit per month.

She certainly is in the "favorable" risk category, so I am proceeding on the assumption that she will be cured. Thank you again for asking us to help look after her. With every best wish.

10

Sanctuary

The second stage of the protocol, known as sanctuary, is designed to seek out possible leukemic cells in the brain and spinal fluid. In Catherine's case this required six medicine-filled spinal taps, three 24-hour hospitalizations for intermediate-dose methotrexate administered by IV, and 8 injections of asparaginase. As we understood the protocol, methotrexate in the normal doses would not cross the blood-brain barrier. However, higher doses would cross over the barrier and kill leukemia cells which might be there. Dr. Truman also told us that in addition to the 24-hour hospital stay we would need to return to the hospital 24 hours after each stay in order for Catherine to be given the "rescue" shot. "Rescue" was the common reference for the drug leucovorin which halted the effects of methotrexate, thereby preventing the high doses from damaging too many healthy cells and causing very serious side effects. In other words you start a time-bomb with the methotrexate and turn it off before it explodes. In the clinic world it was already clear to us that nothing came easily or without some Catch-22.

Over the years many difficult decisions were made. We believe that second-guessing those decisions is not a useful endeavor, and we have accepted the fact that we made judgements based on the best advice and information available to us. Because cancer treatment has evolved over the years it might be tempting to view the past in the light of current information. I believe it was a great strength of our clinic that we were given detailed information, frankly, compassionately, and honestly, and we participated actively in the decision making. We were encouraged to read the available literature and to ask questions, and we were strongly encouraged to keep Catherine and Matthew as informed as their ages and understanding permitted. We believe this approach was the best possible one for our family. Of course we always wondered how this could be happening to our child, but we avoided dwelling on the question, "Why us?" We needed all our strength to deal with day to day living.

The next day after the remission confirmation we were back at the clinic to continue with asparaginase which would be given over the next eight days. One or two doses had already been given in the pre-remission stage. We understood the possible side effects, and in spite of a general uneasiness, we were upbeat and eager to get started in order to get it over with. A complete cart of emergency equipment, including oxygen and a de-fibrillator was standing ready by the treatment cots, as always. We found the presence of the de-fibrillator to be disturbing.

Within thirty seconds of the administration of the drug, Catherine had a severe allergic reaction. It was a nightmare. Her body swelled up like a balloon. She began coughing, choking, complaining of pain in her stomach, and she developed chills and high blood pressure. The symptoms lasted for nearly two hours. Benadryl was administered by IV, an oxygen mask was applied, and she was wrapped in blankets. She looked like a frightened, trapped animal. I remember thinking how tiny the medical equipment was, including the IV needle, the oxygen mask, and the blood pressure cup. Her allergic reaction indicated that asparaginase would not be reasonable chemotherapy for Catherine. This information was recorded in her file immediately and we were instructed to mention it if asked about allergies over the course of treatment.

From Catherine's medical records, October 15, 1980:

Mrs. K. very calm throughout Catherine's reaction. Supportive as well, accepting decision, glad for the rest between meds so family could get their thoughts together. Dad unaware of today's happenings. Monica Corrigan, RN.

From Catherine's dictation, age 6:

Dr. Truman said that I had to take eight asparaginase shots in ten days, but something happened. I had an allergic

reaction. I started throwing up and my body swelled up. I
didn't like it at all. Dr. Truman said, "No more asparaginase
for Catherine—she can live without it!"

On this day while coming home from the clinic after the traumatic afternoon, Catherine and I played the car game of watching the seasons change along the ten mile journey home, especially noting the changes in the woods we passed through. David had invented the game a few days earlier in an attempt to occupy Catherine's mind during the car ride into the clinic for chemotherapy. He correctly surmised that if she was happily occupied it would help relieve the anxiety that she felt. Catherine had acquired a mild fear of foxes (she says from the movie *Bambi*) and we teased each other about where those foxes might be. To this day the drive brings us to the same warm conversation. When we got home we talked and snuggled on the couch, a routine we have all followed over the years. Those conversations in the car going to the clinic and at home afterwards have centered on everyone's feelings about the illness and have helped us sort through all the complexities. The four of us have talked in a group and in all combinations and variations, and at all times of the day and night. Our closeness comes partly from the hours carved out of our lives and devoted to cancer. For David and me, our long, usually late night conversations were complex. I needed to talk a lot and he needed it less. I frequently expressed my frustrations about carrying the burden of the clinic and he countered with the reality of needing to go to work. We were both right. Usually our discussions reached an agreement about how to proceed. When we argued, the disagreement was usually about something we would have argued about at any time of our marriage. Catherine's illness was not a source of conflict for us, although the fatigue and fear it engendered sometimes added a sharp edge. On the other hand, we generally felt that the serious business of managing Catherine's illness made self-centered concerns a luxury we could not afford.

From Matt's college essays, 1991:

My parents handled the situation extremely well, and they
kept their sorrows between them so that we were never

alarmed. We all worked hard in school and at jobs, in spite of difficult times, and we did not give up hope for the success of the treatment. The effect on the family as a whole was to bring us closer together, and my sister and I have remained close.

In the days that followed we prepared for the upcoming first trip to the hospital for the chemotherapy. We organized babysitting, cleared the calendar of responsibilities, and bought little treats for both children which we arranged to give to each of them at the same time. We talked with each about the hospital and about how the family would cope. It was agreed that I would stay overnight with Catherine and David would stay with Matthew.

11

The Hospital

The hospital visit was scheduled for October 23, 1980. Two nights before, as if to remind us how fragile life is, Matthew choked on a piece of meat at the dinner table. He turned bright red, developed a horror-stricken face and tried to talk, but couldn't. As he slowly stood up I heard my own voice saying *Heimlich maneuver* and I went to him and applied the maneuver. I pushed, just as I had seen on TV, and out flew a piece of meat. Matthew started to cry and talk to David and I began to shake and had to leave the room. The whole event seemed to us to fit in perfectly with the general "unreal" feeling that gripped the family as we approached the hospital visit.

Catherine was admitted to the hospital at 11 in the morning. We waited until 7 that evening for the methotrexate to be procured from the pharmacy and the IV to be set up. It was not until after 9:00 that the much feared spinal tap was administered. We were totally unprepared for the delays and despite our best efforts to remain calm, we were upset. Dr. Truman, Dr. Robbins, and Monica came by at 4 p.m. to check on Catherine and keep us apprised of the situation. We expressed our impatience with the delay, but were hesitant to complain out of concern that if we rocked the boat it would come back to haunt us. This is a common fear among parents. David quizzed Dr. Truman about the "rescue" shot scheduled for the following evening at the emergency room. *Would it be too late by the time they got around to us?* Dr. Truman replied: *What! This is not Podunk Memorial Hospital. This is THE Mass. General.* We all guffawed and the tension was eased considerably. Dr. Truman told us that a few hours' delay in the leucovorin is not critical, information that would soon be relevant. David had to head home at 5:30 to take care of Matthew.

Catherine's hospital nurses were a great comfort to her. They stopped by to say hello and they encouraged her to sing: word had traveled that she loved to sing and would do so with the slightest encouragement. They spent time explaining the importance of fluid intake to chemotherapy patients, the seriousness of mouth sores that methotrexate can cause, and the importance of using a prescribed mouth wash regularly. This information had been given during clinic visits, but the repetition was important as there was a great deal of information being given all the time and it was easy to become overloaded. We found over the years that some seemingly small items slipped through the cracks and needed reinforcement. Sometimes Catherine remembered the details better than her parents did! I found the notes in my journal to be very helpful as well.

The spinal tap that night was a disaster. The staff doctor tried three times to insert the needle and finally administered a painful novocaine shot to get the needle in with less discomfort. I held Catherine, who tried desperately to hold still but moved in fear with each stinging attempt. I wondered later if I should have let a stronger person hold her. We finally worked it out. All of us in the small room were perspiring heavily and were exhausted when the procedure was over. Catherine was brave. I believe that the long wait, the sudden blood tests and other surprises, and the rigid hospital routine aggravated what was already a difficult situation. Over the years we learned ways to minimize the impact that hospital regimen had on our lives, but we were green at this time.

From the Journal, October 24, 1980:

A continual problem in the hospital is the complete lack of privacy. This is even hard on a four-year-old. Another problem is the other kids who hang around taking toys, chairs, and liberties with no parent around and no nurses either. Some of the other parents who are there are hard to tolerate. All types of people are to be seen and all are worried, tense, and overdone—just like me. Catherine just seems to withdraw from conversation with all adults including the doctors and nurses. She did tell me in the middle of the night that the doctors and nurses are very nice. We will both be glad to get home.

At 6:45 p.m. on the 24th, Catherine's IV was removed and we were told to head home. Matthew bravely held her hand while she was having the IV removed. At home Catherine had another severe nose bleed and was irritable. We headed into the General on Saturday night for the rescue shot in a blinding rain storm punctuated by flooding and high winds. The drive, which normally took 30 minutes at the height of rush hour, took over an hour. The emergency room staff on duty was the same group from her first hospitalization. They were all glad to see her looking so good, and we were reminded of the need of the staff to see successful outcomes. We were kept waiting for two hours at the emergency room and were told it was because the pharmacy didn't have a supply of leucovorin. Podunk Memorial indeed! In spite of these frustrations, we felt we had with a reasonable degree of success completed the first of the three scheduled trips.

Outside the hospital and the clinic, normal life continued. Halloween came and went, Ronald Reagan was elected by a landslide, we went out to dinner at our favorite restaurant, we raked all the leaves, and Catherine developed mouth sores which were treated and went away.

On November 13, we went back to the hospital. On the way to Boston that morning I experienced what I believe was an anxiety attack (for want of a better word). Literally, I had the feeling that were it not for my skin, my insides would run out all over the place. Strangely, I think I relived in a very brief time the shock of the diagnosis again. Fortunately, the awful sensation passed before we reached the parking lot, and in we went. Again the day was tedious. This time, however, we made arrangements for Matthew so that David could stay during the spinal tap in the hope that his presence would help Catherine. It did. She was much calmer and both the IV and the spinal were uneventful, though painful. Dr. Truman came by and said he wanted to give us the leucovorin kit to take home with us just in case the pharmacy was short or there was another storm. *If you take it home I know it won't get lost!* This thoughtful gesture gave us additional confidence.

In addition to the methotrexate IV, Catherine was given several pints of fluid intravenously during each hospitalization. Commonly she wet the bed several times because of the stupor induced by the drugs and the fluid overload. On this particular occasion the night nurse was intolerant of the problem and hurt Catherine's feelings by calling her a baby. This was said in my presence, and I do not like to think what may have been said by this person to children with no parent in attendance. I complained to the supervisor the next morning, but felt at the time that the complaint was not taken seriously.

Most medical people from doctors to dieticians and from residents to cleaning staff are hard working, dedicated individuals. Occasionally one comes along who should not be doing the job and it does not take too many of those experiences to instill lasting bad feelings in patients and their families. Catherine has never forgotten her feelings of being berated for something she could not help.

From Catherine's 1988 talk to the MGH medical students:

I have told everyone who would listen that it was very hard for me to understand why I wet the bed. I was trying so hard to do what everyone wanted me to do.

To pass the time the next day, we went to the playroom whenever possible. Catherine made pretzels and drew pictures. She missed her brother and sent phone messages to him. He sent her drawings and books and came in to pick her up that evening. That night we went back to the hospital carrying our own leucovorin only to have the staff doctor drop and break the vial. We had to wait an hour for the pharmacy to locate and send another. At home that night Catherine vomited and had a nose bleed.

We passed through the next two weeks trying to recuperate from the hospital experience. Through all the years of Catherine's illness, we noticed that even during the easiest clinic and hospital visits there was a natural recovery time that we needed afterwards. Generally that time was directly proportional to the amount of time spent at the hospital and the severity of the treatment. For example, a brief clinic visit for a small IV might require an hour of recovery time including rest or discussion or silence, while a week in the hospital might mean we took a month or more to return to normal.

We tried to reduce the recovery time to a minimum.

Thanksgiving came and was made wonderful by a visit from my sister Deborah and her family. We all enjoyed good food and good company and the opportunity to talk. During her visit our father became ill in California and we were able to help our parents work out a course of action. It was pleasantly distracting to have one-year-old Daniel in the house and we all found lots of opportunity to laugh and enjoy his antics. At Catherine's clinic visit that week, we were told that we would begin phase three of the treatment, the maintenance phase, which would carry us for the next three years. We also discussed behavior issues with the clinic personnel, including how to separate normal four-year-old behavior from chemotherapy-induced behavior. We have discussed this issue many times since with other parents, and have fully appreciated the sage advice of veteran nurse and mother, Monica. *Discipline is necessary; you won't want a sixteen-year-old who grew up without it.*

On December 4 we went back into the hospital for what we all hoped was the last time. On our way to the ward that day, the MGH social worker pulled me aside to tell me that our little friend Danny had died three days before and had been buried that afternoon with his teddy bear and his match box cars. David and I decided to tell Catherine some other time and to try our best to address the task at hand. The ward staff were devastated by this loss, and the tone of sadness was one we have become accustomed to over the years. Terrible loss is very much a part of the cancer experience. I began reading the obituary column regularly at that time.

The spinal tap that night was done by Dr. Curnutte. With each patient the entry site varies slightly and it is frequently difficult to reach the fluid. When the same person always does the test, that individual becomes familiar with the patient. As yet no one had figured out just how to best approach Catherine. The test took over 30 minutes and left her back with several entry wounds. It was described by our sensitive doctor as *a very rough one.* He had words of praise for her and went out and got her a popsicle for a little treat. She responded well to both things. When we came back for the rescue shot two days later, much to her embarrassment,

Catherine vomited repeatedly in the MGH lobby. About 25 people were in that lobby and only one, an elderly Chinese man, came to our aid. He gave me his handkerchief and asked if he could help us. Words were not enough to express my gratitude to him for caring. Catherine received the rescue IV uneventfully and we closed the book on the hospital phase of the sanctuary stage.

Catherine, age 6:

I remember that I hated having to stay over in the hospital because of the spinal taps.

12

Maintenance

With the hospital behind us, we faced the last two spinal taps the protocol demanded with renewed interest in helping Catherine refine her techniques of pain control and distress management. We showed her the Lamaze breathing techniques we had learned some years before. She learned to concentrate on breathing in a regular rhythm during procedures. She made up stories which she imagined she was in, and she concentrated on peaceful, restful, and enjoyable images. Catherine learned these techniques quickly and was able to reduce her own anxiety during treatment. She called these tricks, getting myself together. Spinal taps 5 and 6, done by Dr. Truman in the clinic, went much more smoothly than those in the hospital, with everyone being supportive and pleasantly surprised at how still Catherine held herself. She took control.

We were eager to meet young people who were surviving cancer and we were introduced to fourteen-year-old Terry on December 15, 1980, a girl from our own town who was ahead of Catherine in treatment, looked wonderful, and who was an all-star tennis player. She and her family seemed happy and self-assured. She spoke cheerfully and optimistically. She was a beacon of hope for us in those early days. In addition to meeting Terry at the clinic, Catherine was thrilled with the new television set which had been donated to the clinic, the first of many donations which we would see come in over the years.

The maintenance phase of Catherine's treatment, designed to kill the small number of remaining cancer cells, was scheduled to last until December of 1983. We were introduced to the schedule, a regimen that included vincristine, methotrexate, 6-mercaptopurine, and prednisone, and were pleased to realize that our clinic visits would be biweekly or even monthly for most of the next two and one-half years if all went well. We felt elated and we moved into the Christmas season with great hope.

From the medical records, December 18, 1980:

Last LP. Catherine and parents very happy. Catherine delightful child. Very cooperative. Brought puppets to clinic for Christmas. Monica, RN.

While the clinic absorbed us, the world lost John Lennon, the hostage situation in Iran went on and on, Chad Green's parents went to court and the charges against them were dropped, Matthew started piano lessons, and my father recovered from a small stroke he suffered over Thanksgiving. We were self-absorbed and needed to be. Christmas was a welcome change, a diversion of great enjoyment. The temperature was 7 below zero and there was snow on the ground. The next morning Catherine began taking daily methotrexate. We felt we were off and running.

On January 5, 1981, the first case of chicken pox was reported at the nursery school and the series of events that ended with Catherine leaving the school unfolded. It was a sad time. Over the years, the chicken pox was a major problem for her. (We have heard that with newly available treatments, chicken pox does not pose the threat today that it did for us.) At her age most of her friends had not had the disease and we all tried to exercise great care. David and I developed a "chicken pox alert" operation to keep track of potential exposures. We wrote a letter of explanation to all parents whose children would come into contact with Catherine asking for a phone call whenever an exposure or a case of chicken pox occurred. The letter worked fairly well and our telephone table soon held lists of callers, exposures, and names of children who were sick, exposed, or immune. The most significant breakdown in this system would come in 1982 when, apparently out of the blue, Matthew would develop the disease and expose Catherine.

During this period of time we settled into the routine that would largely carry us through the next three years. The family occupied most of our free time; both David and I worked long hours at our jobs and we deliberately tried to live as if each day might be the last, while fully expecting to go on forever. We integrated the clinic life into our daily routine, and the people there became part of our extended family. We developed a strong belief in the reliability of the treatment, just as most parents do. We also determined that both children would need some "extras" to lighten up their lives a bit. For Catherine we developed a variety of special treats that were earned by clinic visits. For example, she could choose to make popcorn, pick out a present at the hospital gift shop, order pizza, bake cookies, eat dinner out, or any number of other small tokens. She spent a great deal of time planning the treat. For Matthew we also provided little presents, special notes in his lunch sack, outings to the movies, and eating at his favorite place, the Chinese restaurant. We believed that a positive attitude would be important for maintaining the quality of life we wanted for our family. We also realized that there was some risk of succumbing to the temptation to let go and feel sorry for ourselves, so we discouraged complaining. (Not so easy sometimes.) We insisted that everyone get up on time each morning, clean up, get dressed, and try to face the day cheerfully. Psychologically we wanted to stay optimistic and we believe that our efforts kept us bouyed up, following a philosophy of, *If you get a lemon, make lemonade.* We enjoyed these efforts and they helped.

From the Journal, January 8, 1981:

> *Catherine's blood counts are so high that Dr. Truman has increased her medication to eight methotrexate tablets and one and one-half mercaptopurine. She seems to be doing so well. Dr. Truman says that her condition is no worse than the common cold at present. I love to hear that! They are so upbeat at the clinic—it often feels so good. Imagine laughing at spinals and IVs as if they're nothing. It's terrific.*

The nature of childhood cancer treatment in the 1980s was that all treatment was done in the large established cancer centers. Boston had three such centers while some parts of the country had none, so that some patients had to travel long distances to receive help. We felt fortunate to be in Massachusetts where several choices were available. Each center followed major treatment protocols which have been developed through trial and error over the years and have proven most effective against the disease. Each protocol has some variations of timing and medications designed to allow ongoing comparison, testing, and improvement. In most instances, our clinic used a three year protocol for ALL, while another Boston children's cancer center used a more intensive two year protocol. Both were successful and both were difficult in their own ways. These differences, however, presented some small problems. We found in the small sample of cases in our town that each family had their own unique way of dealing with leukemia that was sometimes influenced by the protocol and certainly by the institution that was administering it. For example, a family whose child was treated at another clinic often reminded us that their child, while getting the shorter treatment, was getting the more aggressive treatment, which they thought was better. This kind of comparison made it difficult to discuss common problems. In addition to appreciating why different protocols are used, we believe that the end results are the important results, not the manner in which they are achieved. In that, most families seem to agree.

During this period, we also heard about cancer treatment from some people we knew and some we didn't. An elderly aunt sent religious treatises which recommended herbal tea and home remedies as the treatment for the whole person. We considered her age, thanked her for caring, and tried to reassure her that we believed we were doing the right thing for our child. Some vitamin salespeople who lived in our neighborhood stopped by the house and pressed us to try the vitamin cure which their company could make available to us for a reasonable fee. I invited them to leave.

Our maintenance routine evolved to one clinic visit per month with daily chemotherapy at home as long as blood counts were strong and illness was not an issue. On February 5, 1981 at our regular clinic visit for vincristine, we met Sue Thompson, the new nurse practitioner. Catherine loved her from the very first day.

From Catherine's English paper, October 31, 1991:

Sue. Her entertaining and lighthearted sense of humor fills the bleak atmosphere with warmth. A hopeful smile and blushing cheeks glow on a pink freckled complexion. Pure blue eyes stare steadily into an ophthalmoscope. A satin-gloved hand grasps another instrument. The movement silkily flows like a ballet dancer. A flowered, pale-blue dress typically hugs the shapely figure, but the straw-gold strands of hair change length unpredictably. A concerned parent asks a question and the tootsie-roll voice gives an answer of wisdom and hope.

From the Journal, March 8, 1981:

March 4 was a clinic day. David went along and read the protocol while we waited. 12B it's called. Soon we go on a new routine. Two weeks on vincristine, three months off. Catherine was very nervous, but she did beautifully. When all was over, she was quite irritable. We had a long discussion in the car going home during which she said she hated leukemia. We told her we didn't like it either and she said, "But you don't have it." Undeniable.

13

Family Days

From the Journal, March 24, 1981:

I think my dear daughter is much affected by her medication since the last increase in dosage. She is extremely irritable and very prone to tantrums. Both of these problems were part of Catherine's behavior before her illness, but now the traits are much exaggerated. Both David and I find her behavior very hard to deal with. We don't know what to do about her distressed state and are trying to hold a firm line and high expectations for her. I feel very self conscious when I try to get her to behave and other people are around. I'm paranoid I guess, but it seems as if people are very critical.

As the much welcomed spring came to New England that year, we were in the throes of trying to understand how to best raise Catherine given the circumstances of her illness and the trauma that was so much a part of her life and ours. We had a deep commitment to following Monica's admonition that discipline was important, yet as young parents we were not altogether certain what was normal four-year-old behavior and what was not. It is clear that it would have been helpful to have a group of parents undergoing similar problems to talk with, but at that time no such group was available at the Mass. General. Since that time, groups have formed and I believe they have been helpful to the families involved. We have been participants and guest speakers at many of them.

Catherine missed her nursery school. She and I devised a plan we called "Catherine's little home school." We planned outings, read books, and did projects regularly. Recognizing that she needed to see other children, we enrolled Catherine in a two day per week nursery school at the local high school in March, and also in a "farm program" in a suburban town near us. As we adjusted to the clinic routine, we were learning quickly how to explain the illness and how to gain assistance documenting the chicken pox exposures in the area. Acting on our instincts and the sound advice of the clinic, we became determined to keep Catherine's life as normal as possible and to expect her to try to overcome whatever difficulties she might encounter. From these early days she learned, like so many of her friends at the clinic, to "tough out" situations that would have sent others to their beds. Sports, drama, art, and academic achievements are the norm for these children, most of whom participate in life to the fullest.

Both Matthew and Catherine began to take swimming lessons at the YMCA in late March. Matt, who had always been fearful of the water, learned to swim strongly and loved it. Catherine was clearly the weakest student in her group, but she enjoyed going with her brother and being with the other children. The Y was very cooperative. We were settling into a rhythmic pattern of activity that I had at one time doubted was possible. Knowing that life could be lived normally was helpful, particularly when events occurred that rocked the boat.

From the medical records, April 29, 1981:

Doing very well though Catherine has been a little more tired in the afternoon recently. Usual dry cough and occasional nosebleeds, but otherwise fine. J. Truman.

From the Journal, May 11, 1981:

Catherine has been complaining of back pains since her swimming lessons today. She has had a very full day and I am hoping that her back is hurting because of fatigue. This illness is full of haunting pains and the bone pain complaint is particularly unnerving. Probably nothing, but if it's not better tomorrow I'll call the clinic.

My sister and her family arrived for another much welcomed visit on May 17. We played cards, went to a Red Sox game, and enjoyed the annual ENKA Fair, a local hospital fundraising carnival. Egged on by his cousins, little Danny, almost two, chanted *EN-KA, EN-KA* all day as we waited to head out to the opening of the fair that evening. At the fair, Catherine developed a nose bleed. I commented to my sister that this was an example of how hard things were and she said, *All kids get nosebleeds.* I retorted, *They don't all get them on a Friday night from drugs taken Friday morning.* I guess I mostly wanted her to agree that my life was hard, whereas she felt obliged to cheer me up and push me to overcome the problems. We observed this pattern with other people at other times: they couldn't be as open about the sadness and hardship as we sometimes needed them to be.

We worried constantly about giving Matthew enough time and attention. We carefully planned special events for him which would give him undivided attention. Matthew during these months was adjusting to first grade and doing well. My journal is full of enthusiasm for his learning to read and other achievements in school:

> *Sweet Boy! Matthew is a bright spot for all of us these days. He is happy and enthusiastic about everything. Today I gave a slide presentation on Winchester history to his class. He was very excited and I am pleased to be able to do something for him.*

Catherine woke up on May 20, 1981 with a fever. Dr. Truman said to take her to her pediatrician who diagnosed pneumonia and prescribed 10 days of amoxicillin. Dr. Keefer indicated that if her fever went up we should call Dr. Truman. We put Catherine to bed and went ahead with the plans for Matthew's seventh birthday on the 21st and Danny's second birthday on the 24th. Matthew was very excited.

From the Journal, May 20, 1981:

> *I can remember clearly the night Matthew was born and now he is seven. He was the most beautiful baby I ever saw. He is still an incredibly handsome boy. Happy Birthday my precious son.*

14

Pneumonia

From the Journal, May 26, 1981:

Only days have passed since I last wrote, but it seems like a lifetime. By Thursday afternoon it was apparent that Catherine was not getting any better. We proceeded with Matthew's birthday party, which Catherine attended wrapped in a blanket and sitting in a lawn chair. She loved being there, but by the end of the party she was fading fast. Her temperature hit 104 degrees. I called Dr. Truman, who said to keep the appointment with Dr. Keefer on Friday. We did and she sent us in to see Dr. Truman at the MGH. Catherine's pneumonia was either viral or pneumocystis, a pneumonia common to immunosuppressed children. Catherine was admitted to the intensive care unit and isolated from other patients. She was placed on oxygen and her arterial blood gasses were measured. Dr. Truman spent 20 minutes with us explaining that we would just have to wait to see what would develop. He said it would get worse before it got better and with his head in his hands he said he did not know how it would go.

This hospitalization was terrifying. Both David and I had the jitters. We couldn't eat and couldn't sleep. We felt totally alone and clung to each other for support. The weekend came and we were left with resident staff doctors, all of whom were competent, but most of whom were strangers to Catherine and to us. The arterial blood gas tests were awful. Normal IVs are inserted in veins near the surface, but the arteries lie deeply hidden under the flesh, and reaching them was a painful ordeal. Catherine was terribly ill, having trouble breathing, pale, and unresponsive. We were asked to wear gowns and masks in her presence, which is frightening to a young child. Coincidentally, the doctor on call that weekend was the same doctor who had sent us out of the room that first night in the emergency room months before. This time he was Catherine's rescuer, and due to his confidence in her improvement and his belief that she would be better off with her parents ungowned, we were allowed to take off the masks and attend to her closely during those critical first two days. When criticized by other doctors for his opinion, he said, *What about her social development?* We were grateful for his deeply felt concern for her welfare.

My sister took care of Matthew for us. She kept the family above water during those few days when we were not sure that Catherine would survive the pneumonia. She stayed until the coast was clear and then went home to California. Late Sunday night after two and a half days in intensive care, Catherine began to show signs of improvement. Three days later Dr. Truman promised that if Catherine could make it through the entire night without the oxygen mask, then we could go home the next day. She did and we did. Over those six days, eleven doctors studied Catherine's case, each asking David and me to recite her history in detail, and all of them examined her, much to her annoyance. At the time we were puzzled by what seemed like an excessive interest in her case. (I think they were looking at all pneumocystis cases in the light of a developing pattern of illness which came to be known as the AIDS epidemic.) But we were so worried about Catherine that we did not give it much thought at the time.

Catherine's story of the hospital stay, December, 1991:

The adult-size oxygen mask I had to wear was far too large for my face and the small mask was for a baby. I felt so sick and bored that all I could do was lie still and watch the television, but the large mask covered my eyes and prevented me from seeing as well as I wanted to. I kept wanting to take it off. I remember this as being a major problem for me and I remember the feeling of that huge mask very well—it felt like I was swallowed up. The small mask was so little it hurt my face and left marks like swim goggles.

From Matt's college essay, Fall 1991:

My life was definitely affected by the whole experience. During her seven years of treatment I was exposed to many things that I would not have known about had Catherine not had leukemia. I can remember holding her hand in the hospital when pneumonia attacked her weakened immune system and brought her close to death.

From a story I wrote after seeing the AIDS Quilt in 1990:

Our family came early to the AIDS issue. In May 1981, our daughter, who was being treated for leukemia, developed pneumocystis carinii and was critically ill. Her treatment with massive doses of Bactrim was accompanied by a tremendous interest by doctors whose specialties were far afield from cancer research. Her primary physician assured us that her illness was related to her reduced immune system resulting from chemotherapy and that these other doctors were only concerned because pneumocystis was showing up in a population other than cancer patients and no one knew why.

In July, 1981, we read a story detailing the newly documented occurrence of pneumocystis carinii in the gay population. From that time on we were tuned in. In early 1982, when some people with hemophilia began to display the same lack of resistance to pneumocystis and other diseases, we learned that there was a possible risk to our daughter because of blood transfusions given to her in September of 1980 when the medical profession was unaware of AIDS.

The standard treatment for pneumocystic pneumonia at that time was large doses of the antibiotic Bactrim. Administered in large doses, Bactrim knocked out the pneumocystis and from that time until six months after she ended chemotherapy in 1987, she took Bactrim daily as a preventive measure. The chest X-rays indicated that her chest would need three to four weeks to clear up completely. On May 29th, two days after her release from the hospital, chemotherapy was resumed.

On May 30th, 1981, David and I celebrated our 12th wedding anniversary and looked forward to summer.

15

Summer

The doctors and nurses at the Pediatric Hematology Clinic were insistent about families living life as normally as possible. They wholeheartedly approved of travel, days off just for fun, and active participation in whatever activities Catherine felt up to doing. We took to this advice like ducks to water! When school ended in June we headed off to New Orleans to visit maternal grandparents and to Tulsa, Oklahoma to check in with paternal grandparents. For both sets of parents, seeing Catherine was heartening, and they began to share our belief that we would get through the treatment successfully.

Getting away from home and from constant reminders of cancer was good for all of us. Along with various relatives we took boat rides and went to the zoo, the amusement park, the Gulf of Mexico, and various shopping malls. All our relatives live outside New England, and we didn't realize before Catherine's illness just how isolated we could be in difficult circumstances. It was helpful to see family even if it was only rarely. Our parents worried about us constantly; in addition to their concern for Catherine, they were worried about us and our welfare. During this visit we realized they needed more reassurance than we did. When one lives every day with a problem one can develop a sense of bravado, of being on the team, so to speak. We actively participated in the treatment as did the children, whereas our relatives could only imagine what was happening, and they often imagined the worst. From that time on we made an extra effort to involve them as much as we could and as much as they wanted and could handle. Their abilities in this regard varied with their own health problems over the long term.

Back in Massachusetts, the chicken pox appeared in the summer and kept Catherine more isolated than she would have wished. We all contented ourselves with enjoying the birth of our friends' baby son on the Fourth of July. We were named his godparents and our children took a great interest in the baby. Tragically, he died of Sudden Infant Death Syndrome on his 27th day and we were plunged back into grief for the loss our friends were suffering. Our friends wondered whether a black cloud hung over our neighborhood.

Catherine was suffering with methotrexate mouth sores at the time and was so miserable that she couldn't eat. We coaxed softened food and ice cream down her and explained again to our children that life can be difficult, but that the measure of man's strength is that he goes on in spite of adversity. Sometimes people asked us how we could go on. They said they could never stand having their child sick with cancer. We didn't really know how to answer them. What were our choices? We frequently said, *How can we give up when Catherine and Matthew face us each night at the dinner table? They depend on us and we can't let them down.* More than just that, however, was the way their youthful enthusiasm carried us along. Already at five and seven, they were no strangers to death and to physical suffering, yet with the resiliency of youth they both laughed, played, sang, and raised the spirits of everyone around them.

Catherine celebrated her fifth birthday with 10 friends and a pool party. She still had mouth sores and was dark-eyed, fatigued, and out of sorts, the result of methotrexate, vincristine, and prednisone. Yet she was thrilled with the birthday attention and happily opened her presents. We marveled that almost a full year had passed, that she had spent 18 days in the hospital, had missed half a year of nursery school, and still had her hair!

We headed off for our annual pilgrimage to Bar Harbor, Maine, and Acadia National Park, and enjoyed some great swimming, hiking, and eating. On our third day there, Catherine awoke with a fever, aching hip joints, and more mouth sores. Chemotherapy kills some normal cells along with many cancer cells, and the white blood cells of the immune system originating in the bone marrow were among the most susceptible. By now we recognized the signs of low blood counts and began watching the fever. By the next morning, she had a fever of 101 degrees and we called the clinic for advice and prepared to head home. Seven hours later at the clinic her blood counts were in and the news was not so good: a low red cell count and a white count of only 800. Her platelet count remained in the normal range. (Our understanding was that a low platelet count would suggest also a possible resurgence of leukemia cells.)

The clinic personnel did not jump to place their young patients in the hospital if it could be avoided, so we went home to rest with the admonition that if her fever went to 102, she would be admitted. Twenty-four hours later in the emergency room after five attempts at inserting an IV, Catherine was started on broad spectrum antibiotics to help protect her while her immune system recovered.

From the medical record, August 14, 1981:

> *Platelet count normal—very reassuring that this episode of neutropenia and anemia is due to chemotherapy suppression of marrow. She has been taking adult-size doses of 6MP and MTX to date with only minimal marrow suppression—no surprise that this is at last catching up with her. John Truman.*

From the Journal, August 15, 1981:

> *Catherine slept fairly well last night. She is quite irritable, but is smiling and watching cartoons. She is complaining about pain surrounding her IV. It may not last and she is quite fearful. Our roommates are quite interesting; bone cancer, a broken back, and colitis. Catherine is the youngest and likes being with the older girls. We are exhausted. This is no picnic.*

After four days, Catherine's counts were returning to her normal level (still low by healthy child standards) and she was feeling well enough to get up, go to the playroom, and visit her six-year-old friend Susie who was in the final stages of her illness and was not expected to live much longer. (Susie had suffered the same type of relapse that Catherine was destined to face two years later.) Catherine cheerfully talked to her friend, who couldn't speak any more, and Susie seemed happy to have her visit. Her parents were sitting on the bed playing a board game and talking with the girls. Their bravery was typical of parents in their situation. They made every minute count. After we left Susie's room, Catherine commented that she was sorry her friend couldn't talk with her because she usually loved to talk. At the time, I thought that Catherine did not really know what was happening. Nine years later, in freshman English class, Catherine wrote this poem.

Susie

I shuffled through the bleached white corridor
A cold brown door loomed, open
She hovered like an angel on her bed
A curtain of grey shadows advancing.

Here my friend sat
Her face colorless and shallow as a cloud
She wanted to speak
But her words had been stolen away.

Life to us was pills and needles
Merely four, I only half realized
Her cancer was determined
To seize her life too.

The next morning Catherine's long blond hair began to fall out by the handful. Perhaps it was the chemotherapy, perhaps the fever, perhaps the low blood counts. We trimmed what was left to shoulder length and cut bangs to make it look like it covered her head. She sobbed briefly and bravadoed her way through it. We started calling her *toughie*. She was released on August 19 and we began to regroup at home.

Every hospital stay was difficult. The family was separated, the sleeping arrangements for parents at the hospital were almost non-existent, and the facility was old with few bathrooms and either too much heat or too much air conditioning depending on the time of year. There were always heart-breaking situations with some of the other children that quietly raised the tension level for both staff and parents. We learned over the years that we had to be advocates for our child and that sometimes what we felt to be in her best interest was out of sync with hospital procedure. Not too surprisingly we developed a bit of a reputation among some of the staff nurses and doctors, but, in general, I believe they supported our efforts. We know Catherine benefited from having at least one of us there with her all the time and that the frequent visits of her brother and some selected friends were helpful. Whenever she was hospitalized, the clinic staff visited her twice a day. For all the years that Catherine was on treatment, every hospital stay took an additional toll on all of us.

From the Journal September 1, 1981:

I have been having a very hard time the last few weeks. Once again, going to the hospital and the fear attached to it is very hard to shake off. With kindergarten starting next week we had to explain the chicken pox issue to the school and write a letter to all the parents letting them know the situation and asking them for help. It is very painful to be unsure as to whether or not they will call us. Our experience with getting help on this issue has not been so good.

Despite the ups and downs of the summer of 1981, we headed into the school year ready to go and hopeful for a good beginning for each child. To introduce the school and parents to Catherine's situation we sent the first of a long series of "chicken pox letters" to her classmates' families.

Sept. 8, 1981

Dear Parents,

We are the parents of Catherine Krumme who will be a classmate of your child in the kindergarten at Lincoln School. Catherine has leukemia and is undergoing chemotherapy. She has had this condition for one year and has two years of treatment left. The chemotherapy leaves Catherine's immune system in a depressed state. This causes her few problems with regard to childhood illnesses with the exception of the chicken pox. We are asking for your help in this regard. We need to minimize the risk to Catherine while at the same time we want her to have as near normal school attendance as possible.

We have two defenses against chicken pox. First, if a child has been exposed to chicken pox, we will keep Catherine from coming in contact with that child during the time that the disease might be contagious. (We consider this time to be between 7 and 21 days after exposure, although the most likely time is 14 days.) And second, if Catherine is exposed, she can be given a serum which if given within 48 hours of exposure will control the disease. (Fortunately, the disease is contagious for no more than 24 hours before the spots show, so it is always possible to know of an exposure in time to get the serum.) If both these measures fail and Catherine gets the chicken pox, she will likely get very sick with it.

What we need from you is that you notify us immediately if your child comes down with chicken pox or if you think she or he may have been exposed to it. We can then decide what should be done and take the necessary steps to protect Catherine. Chicken pox is the only disease we need to take special precautions for; Catherine has no problem with exposure to colds, flu, or any other common illnesses. If you have any questions, please feel free to call us.

We are looking forward to a happy kindergarten experience for our daughter and she is looking forward to new friends and "real" school.

Thank you for your cooperation.

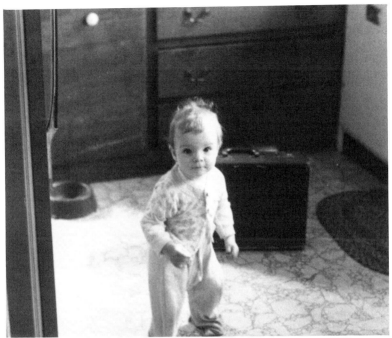

Catherine began walking at eight months in April 1977.

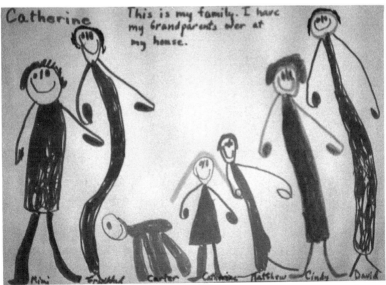

Catherine's nursery school drawing of her family was made the day she was released from the hospital after her initial diagnosis in September 1980.

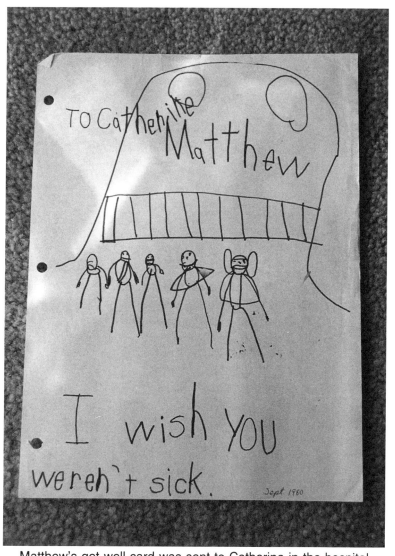

Matthew's get-well card was sent to Catherine in the hospital in September 1980.

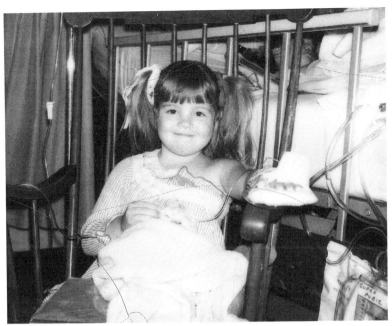

Catherine, age four, mugged for her family during one of three hospitalizations for intermediate dose methotrexate. October 1980.

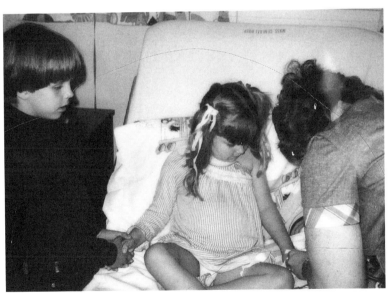

Matthew, age six, helped Catherine get her IV removed in order to go home. October 1980.

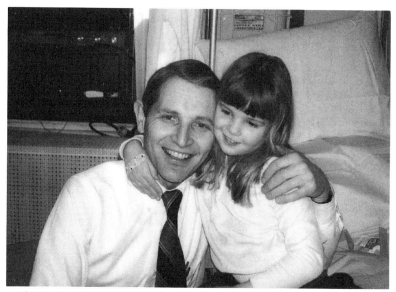

Catherine felt comfortable with "her Dr. Truman." March 1981.

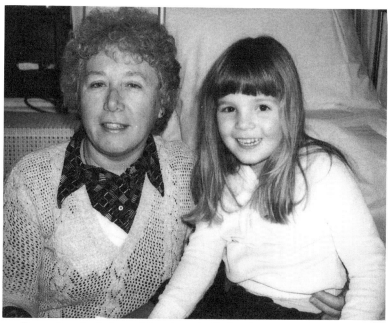

From the first day of treatment, Catherine spent hours with Monica. March 1981.

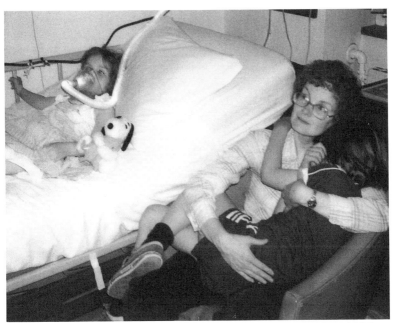

Catherine's bout with pneumocystic pneumonia in May 1981 took an emotional toll on the family just as each hospital stay did. She hated the oxygen mask.

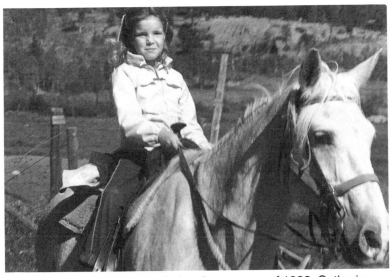

At the ranch in Colorado during the summer of 1983, Catherine felt in control of "Snowball."

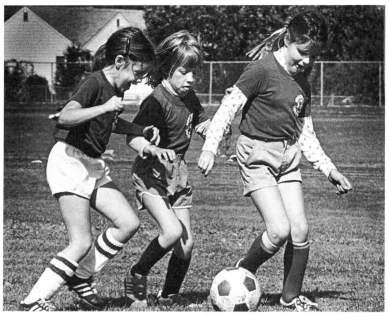

Catherine began playing soccer. She enjoyed all aspects of the game, which she played through the ninth grade, but mostly she enjoyed being with her friends.

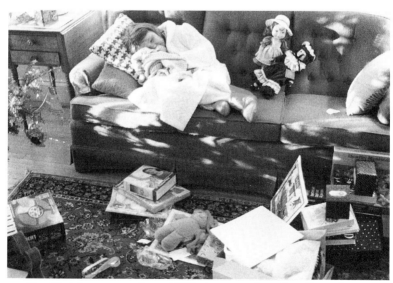

On Christmas morning, 1983, four weeks after the relapse, Catherine fell asleep right after opening gifts.

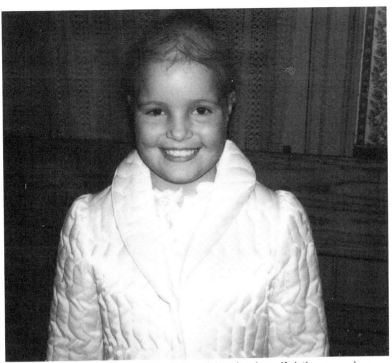

Catherine's hair began to fall out by the handful the morning after Christmas. Her round cheeks show the water retention caused by steroids.

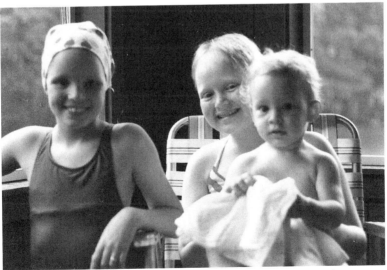

Catherine and Lauren (holding her nephew) smiled together on the day they floated in the pool. This is the last photo of the girls together.

Clinic Rules

1. Must have a good sense of humor.
2. Must always do a good LP, B.M.
3. Must always remember the toy box.
4. Must tell the truth to anyone who wants it.
5. Must like people.
6. Must like junk food.
7. Must know a lot about chemotherapy.
8. Must not mind the sight of blood.
9. Must like bald heads.
10. Must never be grumpy.

Catherine's clinic rules were handwritten in the car on the way to Boston. They were kept posted on the wall at the clinic for years.

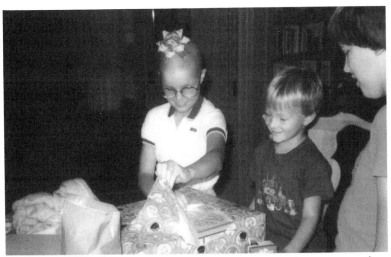

Catherine, cousin Danny, and brother Matthew opened presents at her eighth birthday party. With no hair, she stuck the package bows to the top of her head.

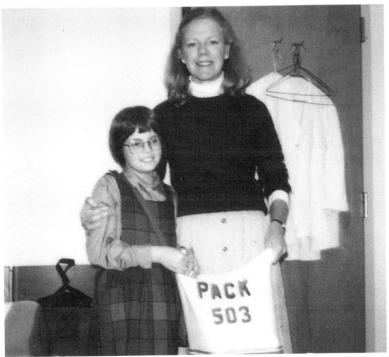

Cub Scout Pack 503 began sending toys to the clinic in 1984. Catherine and Sue played Santa Claus. Catherine is wearing her wig.

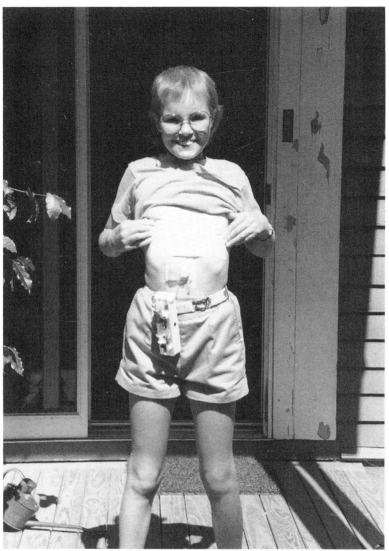

Catherine shows off the pump! She hated the pump but was proud of her new hair.

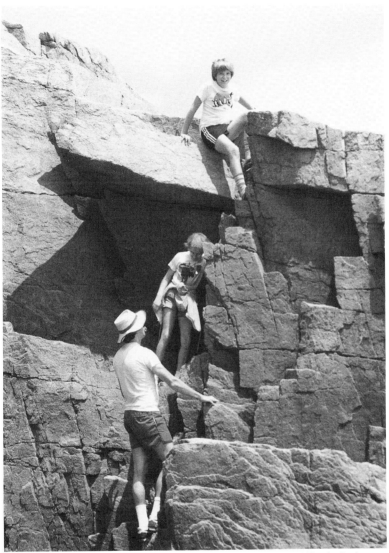

The family began rock climbing at Acadia National Park during the summer of 1985.

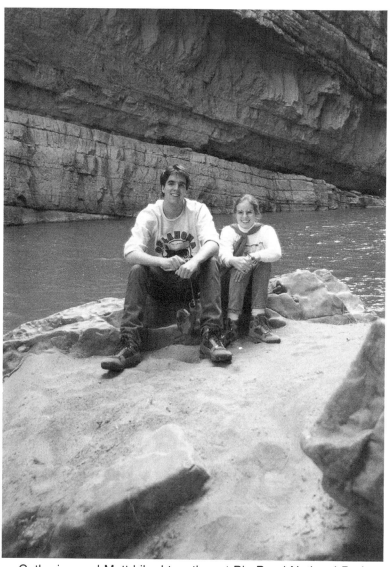
Catherine and Matt hiked together at Big Bend National Park in February of 1991.

16

Settling In for the Long Haul

Catherine began her kindergarten year with great enthusiasm. She reveled in the opportunity to be with other children and looked forward to learning new things. The class had 27 students and the teacher worried about the size of the class and the presence of a child with cancer. We tried to reassure her. An irony that we felt and others expressed was that the difficulty of living with cancer is sometimes compounded when much of the reassuring must come from the patient and the family toward the rest of the world.

Just after school started Catherine's friend Susie died. We took her death hard, and we found that most of our friends and family seemed unable to talk with us about it. Catherine and Matthew both asked about Catherine's leukemia and we all tried to reassure each other. Two weeks later, another six-year-old friend, Paul, lost his fight. He had bravely shown Catherine how to survive an IV without crying and she struggled to live up to his example. After hearing the news of Paul's death, Catherine curled up on the couch with me and asked if all children died from leukemia when they were six. We have made it our practice to talk openly among ourselves about the children we know from the clinic, but as the years went by and the losses piled up, we found it easiest not to mention our clinic friends to our hometown friends very often. For the most part we kept our grief within our family.

Catherine, dictated at age 6.

In the beginning, I had to go to the clinic a lot to get

vincristine. One of those days at the clinic I met a friend named Paul. He taught me how not to be scared from an IV. He was very brave because he had had so many of them. I used to see Paul at the clinic a lot. About a year later Paul got sick and died. I felt very sad.

From the Journal, September 1981:

Only Susan and Bill and Judy and Paul seem to be able to listen to us talk about cancer without changing the subject. We sometimes feel very lonely and isolated.

After the intensive visit schedule during the preceding months, we settled back into the routine of monthly clinic visits. Generally Catherine and I would go in after school. The car ride took about 30 minutes and allowed us time to chat, prepare mentally for the treatment, and make up games to pass the time. Whenever possible, David took off work to go with us, and Matthew frequently came along to take care of Catherine. Over the year, both children experienced some regression in behavior, some sleeping problems, and some general irritability. Independent Matthew became clingy, and tough little Catherine hugged her blanket and took her teddy bear Freddy everywhere. We observed that they both were able to talk about how they felt and to express rather clearly, considering their ages, their feelings about what was happening. David and I were having similar problems. Sleeping was sometimes difficult and we spent most of our free time together talking about leukemia and our children. Only when the years passed and treatment ended did we fully realize just how much time and energy we both put into getting Catherine well.

We decided that fall that it would be helpful to find a group of parents of children with cancer. MGH still had no support group for us and we looked around at our options. Our local hospital had a cancer support group for patients' family and friends and they said we could come. Only two of the families had a child with cancer, and the needs of adult patients and children are somewhat different. We did profit from meeting the other families, but we only went to that group twice.

From the Journal, October 30, 1981:

The other parent of a child with leukemia in the group announced that of course his son and my daughter were at different clinics getting different treatment and that that kept our families apart because each one needed to believe that his or her treatment was the best. I said that we didn't feel that way, but I felt out of place in the group after that.

Different people react differently to cancer. We learned that some families do well and some do not. Separation and divorce are common among clinic families, but frequently there were strains in the marriage before the cancer. In our experience, cancer alone was not the cause for the breaking up of families. Nonetheless, the families where the marriages split apart suffered a great deal. It is hard enough to live with cancer when everyone is pulling together. Both David and I were in our early 30s when Catherine became ill. We had been married for 11 years and had known each other since high school. We had an adequate income, health insurance that took care of all the bills, and we accepted each other's different ways of dealing with our hurt and worry. We struggled to express our concerns and to keep each other informed in as constructive a way as possible concerning our needs and the needs we felt for our children. Every day Catherine and Matthew looked at us expectantly across the breakfast table and we hung in there for them and for ourselves.

One and a half years after Catherine's diagnosis, the MGH began a group for parents of children in our clinic. We went for six months. We believe that a well-run group is worthwhile, especially in the early days of treatment when everyone is struggling to learn the ropes. Other parents who have been at it for a while are a gold mine of practical information. We couldn't wait to talk to the parents of children who were almost done, or who were off treatment. We eagerly took in any information we could get regarding successful treatment. We sought out examples of young people who were doing well, who were staying in school, who were active and learning and living life to the fullest in spite of their cancer. We found those parents and children everywhere and they became our beacons. At the same time, after a year and a half we were old timers already and were frequently asked questions by the newcomers. Repeating the wonderful advice given me in the first days, I recommended keeping a journal to everyone who asked me any question at all.

In December of 1981, our clinic moved from its too-small, too-cozy space in the old MGH to its austere new space in the new outpatient building. The new clinic shared its waiting room with several other clinics and we felt a loss of privacy and closeness that we had enjoyed in the previous location. However, within weeks "our kids" had taken over most of it, and harmony reigned.

From the 1981 Christmas letter:

> *I am happy to report that we are all doing well and feeling good. Catherine is now five and in her 16th month of treatment for leukemia. The initial remission has lasted and the prognosis is excellent. We still have two years of treatment and then four more years until they will pronounce a cure. We continue to be sure that she has the best possible chance. The past year has been eventful, happy, sad, difficult, and easy some of the time. We take the days one at a time.*

Over the course of the Christmas holiday, Catherine developed hand and foot tremors from vincristine and began to experience severe nausea. Her doctor reduced her dosage slightly, which offered enough relief that she could take the rest of it cheerfully. The tremors made her somewhat unsteady, and the response of the public school was to ask us to sign a waiver releasing them from liability if she fell or was hurt at school. We refused on principle and they did not press the issue. To us, the risk of injury from falling down was negligible compared with pneumocystis, low blood counts, cancer, and so on. The school's response was somewhat typical in that they acted in extreme ways to most problems, and they considered having a child with cancer in the school to be a serious problem. We found that how Catherine was treated at school depended largely on the support of the principal. Until 1984, she went to a school with a principal who considered her presence there to be a problem.

In January 1982, we delighted in the realization that with one year of a remission under "maintenance" chemotherapy under our belts, Catherine's chances for recovery were much improved. We found it slightly easier to feel and project confidence. January and February brought several cases of potential chicken pox exposure. For a child who loved school as much as Catherine did, this was sometimes as difficult as being sick. We had to struggle to keep her in touch with friends and up to date with school work. Throughout her years of treatment it was difficult to keep friendships going. She was either not there, too tired to play, too sick to join in, or too emotionally drained to care. Catherine learned to play alone and to depend on her imagination. She enjoyed singing, making up little shows with her dolls, and painting pictures by the hour. Her brother spent hours of his own free time teaching her soccer, playing board games, and keeping her company. He took this role seriously and he is still her closest friend.

In late February, chemotherapy made her blood counts dip dangerously low again, this time her platelet count as well as her hematocrit and white blood count, and she developed a high fever. Catherine spent seven more days in the hospital on IV antibiotics while her counts recovered. We were unaware at the time just how concerned the clinic was by the platelet count; they worried that it might indicate problems (cancer) in the bone marrow.

From the medical records, February 18, 1982:

> *If counts do not rise within next four to five days we should look at her bone marrow. May now be allergic to penicillin. Hives at IV site—no recurrence when given Bactrim. J. Truman.*

Fortunately, her counts gradually went up and she was released. She finally was able to go back to school after missing nearly one month between the hospital and the chicken pox cases. By this time our chicken pox network was very complete. Our friends kept alert and reported any rumored outbreak to us, and the school notified us every time they were notified by any family in any class. (Matthew had not had the disease either, so our vigilance was applied to both children.) We thought that if the government wanted to track the course of chicken pox through eastern Massachusetts, it need only ask us for our records.

17

Chicken Pox

Matthew broke out with chicken pox at school where it was observed by his teacher. I was at a meeting and not available by phone so our friend Judy was called and she took him home. I got the message at three in the afternoon. Unbeknownst to anyone, he had been exposed and he had now exposed not only his entire class, but his sister as well. It was ironic that we missed both the exposure and the onset of the symptoms!

After picking up Catherine and calling the clinic to arrange for the V-ZIG (a protective shot of varicella zoster immune globulin administered in each leg), I went to Judy's to see him briefly and to reassure him that everything would be alright. Although he was not feeling well, he was being brave and I left him in the loving hands of our friend.

Catherine was terrified! The chicken pox had been a hidden terror to her. It had kept her out of school, caused her to miss activities, and she was aware that it could be very dangerous if she were to get it. Her nurse Sue held her in her arms and reassured her that the ZIG combined with skipping all chemotherapy for two weeks would keep any case she might develop from being too serious. She also told her that the ZIG was painful and that she was terribly brave. The shots were given into the muscle of both thighs, with Catherine holding my hand and looking with trusting eyes at her dear Sue.

We knew that some children undergoing chemotherapy at our clinic had died from the chicken pox, and from our perspective at the time this was one of the worst things that could happen to her, next to a relapse. We were also uneasy about skipping chemotherapy for a period of time that might extend into a month if she actually came down with the chicken pox. We went home to wait it out and take care of Matthew.

Matthew was relegated to the position of Typhoid Mary. In our big old house we were able to isolate him from Catherine by moving him into the guest room which has its own bathroom. We set him up with the television and assorted games, toys, and presents. The guest room is directly above the kitchen so he was able to pound on the floor when he needed more food. Since he was feeling reasonably well—he only developed 20 pox during the entire illness—this arrangement developed into a delightful game. Once walkie-talkies were added with which he could call Catherine or us in any part of the house, he actually controlled the house. By the end of the week he was chomping at the bit and Catherine was trying to sneak as close as possible to his room in order to *see Matty* and keep him company. He also had a steady stream of visitors who had already had the chicken pox.

As it turned out, the boy who sat next to Catherine in her class came down with the chicken pox the next day, so if she had not had the ZIG from the exposure to her brother, then she would have had it the next day. In all, she missed three more weeks of school waiting for the disease to run through her classmates. Much to everyone's surprise, Catherine never developed the chicken pox in spite of this close exposure.

From the Journal, April 5, 1982:

Still no recognizable chicken pox. The last three weeks have been very difficult. We would really like to see one little spot that we could recognize as chicken pox so we would know she would be protected in the future from other exposures. We must wait two months to test her immunity.

From the Journal, June 6, 1982:

We had Catherine tested for chicken pox immunity and she did not have any. This is very disappointing as we had hoped that she had a very light case perhaps. Nothing has really changed, but we were very hopeful of having some of the burden lifted. There is still so much chicken pox around.

Now there are so many exposures in Catherine's class that she must leave school on Tuesday for the duration of the year. What a complicated existence!

During the year that followed, Catherine participated in the National Chicken Pox Immunization Study. She was vaccinated, not once, but twice. Her little three-year-old cousin Danny bravely donated three blood samples as the control family member. The second vaccine seemed to work and gave us over a year free from worry. In the final blood sample taken for the study, one year after Catherine's relapse, it appeared that her vaccine-acquired immunity (titer) had disappeared. We managed to keep her away from others with the chicken pox, and as she grew older that became easier since most of her friends had had the disease already. We were surprised and remain amazed at how few people are aware of the serious nature of the chicken pox virus. Not only is the disease serious for immunosuppressed people, it carries some risk to healthy individuals as well. At the time Matthew had the disease we knew of a child in town who was so covered with pox that she was hospitalized for breathing problems.

18

Mountains

The summer got off to a rocky start for Catherine. Her blood counts were unstable, preventing her from getting her regular chemotherapy. Not being able to get chemotherapy was always upsetting.

June was rainy, which seemed appropriate. Catherine missed the last month of school due to chicken pox in her class. While she was unhappy not to be in school, Matthew couldn't wait to get out of school. David was working hard to establish his academic career as he would be considered for tenure in the next year and he was concerned that the time constraints and strain that leukemia had placed on him might have impacted his work too much, thereby weakening his tenure case. Not just a job was at stake: we were concerned about keeping our health insurance. I was spending much of my time working with Catherine to help her keep up in school and considering various job possibilities for myself. During this time I decided that I would not return to my job as a public school teacher and instead would make a career change when the time for returning to work became apparent.

In July the weather improved drastically and so did Catherine's blood counts. We took our annual trip to Bar Harbor, with Catherine feeling strong enough to swim daily and take short but strenuous hikes. We had to leave Maine a day early because she suddenly developed a fever and we felt it advisable to head home just in case it turned into another hospital visit. At the clinic that week we heard that the bone marrow transplant of one of our little friends had gone well. Louie had been diagnosed with the same form of leukemia the same week as Catherine and over the years we had developed a friendship with him and his mother. We enjoyed and profited from our clinic alliances. We were exposed to the ups and downs of the families we knew and we shared their joys as well as their sorrows. Clearly the parents learned from talking to each other and sharing experiences. We were a lot like family to each other. As we expected, Catherine's counts were not good enough for chemo-therapy that week, but her fever went away on its own.

From the Journal, July 28, 1982:

A resident doctor on his brief rotation through the clinic pointed out to us that the high counts (an early indicator of a relapse) *were probably not her cancer coming back. She understood what he was implying and was alarmed. We had not considered the possibility of cancer and we knew more about the meaning of the blood counts than he did. Next week we are going to the afternoon clinic so we will avoid the crowds of amateur hematologist/oncologists on rotation. Perhaps I'm cheating future doctors of contact with our girl, but it will spare her such comments.*

That August we celebrated Catherine's sixth birthday and the birth of a new baby girl next door. Born into the family who had lost their son the summer before, her arrival was heralded. Because her older sibling had died of SIDS, she was placed on a monitor which would buzz loudly if her breathing patterns were disturbed in any way. Despite the inconvenience of the device and its continual reminder of the previous loss, she thrived and brought joy to everyone. Catherine was particularity intrigued with the baby as she was viewed as old enough to help out.

In late August we made our first trip to Colorado to the Long's Peak Inn and Guest Ranch just outside Rocky Mountain National Park. The family style ranch was an excellent change for us. The hiking and horseback riding gave both children a chance at independence. They were able to strike off with the ranch staff to ride all day, hike, sleep out in a teepee, and we can only guess what other activities! The nature of treating cancer in children over such a long time is that they are forced to be dependent on parents and doctors. Frequently, the way they feel keeps them from breaking away both physically and emotionally. The Ranch experience, with its independent activities and its great beauty in the Rockies, opened up a whole new world to all of us and we have gone there every summer since, except for the summer after the relapse. For months after, whenever the time permitted, the children played "dude ranch" with little plastic animals and people.

From the Journal, August 1, 1991:

Catherine climbed Long's Peak: sixteen miles up and back, 14,255 feet of elevation. She can do anything! Who would have ever thought it possible? When we first came to Colorado, she needed help to walk a half mile.

Back home in early September, 1982, Catherine developed a nagging chest cold and a red itching rash on her hands and feet. The rash, never diagnosed, remains a mystery to us, just another in a long steady stream of slightly bizarre reactions that she had over the years. In retrospect, it seems that Catherine often came home from travel with colds, strange rashes, and general fatigue; but she also came home with the belief that she was just like everyone else. She took vacations, she worked hard, she played hard, and she delighted in life most of the time. We never considered giving up travel, we just followed the clinic's advice about how to minimize infections, get enough rest, and live to the fullest. The way we saw it, if she was going to survive the cancer, there was no reason she should miss out on three years of life during the treatment, and if she was not going to survive it, she had to pack a whole lifetime into those years. Either way, it was a time to maximize her involvement in the world. Some people supported us in these decisions and some thought we were crazy.

19

Time Marches On

The start of Catherine's first grade year was the same as the end of her kindergarten year. She had to miss the first two weeks of school due to chicken pox in her class. When she finally went to school she was off and rolling. She established a good relationship with her talented teacher, just as her brother had done the previous year. With the encouragement of the clinic, she started playing Saturday morning soccer in the town recreational league.

Catherine and Matthew traded cases of the flu back and forth for a major part of the fall and winter. Matthew continued to have the frequent ear infections he had had since infancy. Surgically implanted tubes at age four had helped, but he still had the tendency to develop infections. David and I began to re-establish ourselves in our activities outside work and cancer treatment, and in general we began to relax. We found we were able to listen with envy to descriptions of treatment that ended in two years rather than three. While we were not interested in changing the treatment, we were eager for it to be over, for the three years to pass, and for our lives to return to the pre-cancer days. I believe that such thoughts were a sign that our confidence was growing.

From the Journal, September 1982:

> *Dr. Truman told us today that in England they use the MGH protocol that Catherine is on, only they quit the treatment after two years and they get the same results. Very intriguing.*

On November 15, 1982, our clinic was featured on a Boston television station and we were introduced by the program to a wonderful girl named Lauren whom we later came to know well. The following week we filed for a tax number for a small business endeavor in software marketing through which we hoped to finance some parts of two college educations.

Overall, the visits to the clinic throughout the second year of treatment had been less stressful for us in terms of time and frequency, but they took their toll on Catherine whenever she got chemo. Our lives were still governed by the clinic and the treatment.

From the Journal, November 26, 1982:

Catherine got her vincristine on Wednesday and she is suffering a bit. Her skin color is sallow and her eyes are sunken and dark. The prednisone is beginning to make her body swell and she has cried on and off for two days. In spite of this she had a great Thanksgiving.

From the 1982 Christmas letter:

Greetings from springlike Massachusetts. This year is more like Christmas in Berkeley! We are all doing well and keeping busy. Six-year-old Catherine is only 12 months away from the end of chemotherapy. We will be happy to see the end of daily drugs and frequent IVs. She is as terrific as ever. We have very much appreciated everyone's kind thoughts and loving understanding. Eight-year-old Matthew is a third grader. After all the time I spent teaching third grade, it is amazing to me that I have a child that age! Both children continue to grow like weeds and both continue to delight and amaze us with the things they do and say in the course of a day.

So another year has passed and we find ourselves in good spirits—still taking life one day at a time.

From the Journal, December 17, 1982:

The New York chicken pox people report that Catherine has a titer! The vaccine worked this time and she has some immunity. I hope the study people realize that there is a real six-yearold girl on the other end of the blood tubes and that this is a very important piece of news for her.

We had a wonderful Christmas. In early January, Catherine started taking piano lessons, something she had especially wanted to do. Just before Christmas, the clinic had received a big toy box from the Charley Davidson Leukemia Fund which had been set up the previous December in memory of a little boy who had died in 1981. The toy box was kept brim-full of toys, books, and tapes for children of all ages. The rules for getting into the box were that you had to have a "significant" procedure of some kind, not just an IV. As we would come to know, some children got to get into the toy box a great deal. At this point in time, Catherine was a little envious of those who got to use it, and she looked forward to the end of her treatment when the requisite spinal tap and bone marrow would allow her to look inside the box. In addition, the fund bought a VCR, and tapes arrived which we made the most of to pass the time on treatment days. We were delighted when the fund was established. It gave us something to suggest to distant family and friends who asked what they could do to help. The fund furnished the clinic with many amenities it had not had before.

The winter of 1983 was cold and snowy. We enjoyed the snow days—no school—but by late March we were ready for a change. Over the winter and into spring, the various combinations of Catherine's drugs affected her in different ways. The treatment strategy was to give her the maximum dosage that her system could tolerate without crashing her blood counts completely. The consequence of this strategy was that dosages were being altered at nearly every visit. We worked hard at not anticipating reactions, because sometimes they didn't materialize and we wished to remove the component of fearful expectation from the equation. Throughout that entire third year, no other medication had the impact on her that vincristine and prednisone did. We eagerly looked forward to the end.

From the Journal, March 21, 1983:

> *Catherine has made it through another two weeks of prednisone and vincristine. She was pretty miserable much of the time: tiredness, insomnia, starving all the time, pain in her legs and hips and very weepy. She is very strong and tries to be cheerful. It is very hard to bear for her and for us all.*

From the medical records, April 6, 1983:

Catherine continues to do well. She loves school and every-thing in general and is doing just fine. Sue Thompson, RN.

In May, 1983, David was awarded tenure at Tufts University. I had been worried about tenure because we needed to stay near the Mass. General for Catherine's sake. Tenure added a measure of security to our lives that we needed. David and I both felt relief and a sense of accomplishment.

At ages six and nine, both Catherine and Matthew were happy-go-lucky children. They liked school, enjoyed sports, had friends, and behaved in an age-appropriate manner most of the time. However, in one way they differed from most children their own age: they saw death regularly.

From the Journal, May 15, 1983:

Today I helped in Catherine's Sunday School class. They were talking about death and grief and she brought in a picture of Susie to share with the other children. She told them she didn't know any cats or dogs who have died—only people. It was very sad to hear her tiny little voice talking about dead friends. (When Catherine was in the fifth grade, her Sunday School class again had a unit on death and grief. She wouldn't attend the classes, because she said the children didn't take it seriously and she wasn't going to try to explain it to them anymore.)

On May 23, 1983, four-year-old Louie died after a long struggle. It was a painful time for us all. Catherine told us that she was sometimes afraid that she would die too, and even Matthew, who always talked about Catherine being well, asked if it was possible that she might die. On May 29, 1983, we proudly watched as one of David's students received his Bachelor's Degree. He developed leukemia at the age of 13 and was then 23. Our lives were full of contrasts.

From Meredith, a young friend, to Catherine, May 24, 1983:

I am sorry that your friend died. I know you must be feeling sad, because it is hard to lose someone you like so much. If you are feeling sad and you would like to be with a friend I hope you would come over to my house and we could be together and play church or dress up or something. I hope you feel better.

From Matt's college essay, 1991:

She received her chemotherapy at a clinic for childhood cancer, a place that we frequently visited and that is engraved in my memory. I saw other children who, like my sister, were struggling against leukemia. I learned to deal with death because many of those children died from the disease. I never believed that Catherine wasn't going to make it and I viewed myself as her partner, whose job it was to help her.

The First Last Six Months

In June 1983, nurse Sue told us that the schedule would bring us to the end of treatment in late November. We were pleased to think ahead to that time and interested in keeping our activities at a normal level. I had started volunteering with the local cable TV station and was enjoying producing, writing, and taping local programs, and I spent most of my disposable free time doing just that. That summer I began teaching video production at the town recreation department, in addition to managing our off and running software company.

Working with Sue, we had detailed a treatment schedule that would place most of Catherine's heavy duty chemo on Friday afternoon so that during the school year she would have the benefit of the weekend to recuperate. Our clinic schedule allowed us to be away for two full weeks and we took advantage of the time whenever possible. In July we took off to visit grandparents once again and this time drove from Louisiana through Texas to Oklahoma. While in Oklahoma we visited my younger sister Rebecca, who had Down's Syndrome and lived most of her adult life in a home in Okmulgee, Oklahoma. I had not seen her in two years and wanted to very much.

From the Journal, August 3, 1983:

> *Today Catherine celebrated her seventh birthday. This is very significant for us as this is the year that her treatment ends and we can see a girl without pills and IVs. Hooray! I don't believe she will ever have a birthday that we aren't grateful to see. David thinks a lot of people feel that way!*

We went back to "our" Colorado ranch for a second year. Catherine fully participated in their riding program and spent most of every day out on a horse with "her wrangler friends." She was feeling strong in part due to a reduced medication schedule because of low blood counts again. Dr. Truman insisted that we go ahead with the planned trip. His go-for-it attitude was based on his philosophy of treating the whole child and in our case he knew full well that the whole family benefited from the trips we took. The logistics of travel were sometimes complicated, but the rewards were great. We didn't yet know how easy things were, compared to what they could be.

Catherine started second grade on time with her class with no chicken pox worries for the first time. We began to plan for the end of treatment and we enthusiastically built up our expectations. We believed that the leukemia was gone and that the treatment had already been successful, so we concerned ourselves more with chemotherapy-related illness than with cancer itself.

From the Journal, September 26, 1983:

> *For some reason I have remembered all morning all the times we have almost lost her. She is awfully young to have the kind of track record she has. My main worry now is that her chemo will make her sick again.*

In October we decided to participate in the Charley Davidson Leukemia Fund Walkathon which was held in the neighboring town of Lexington. Our local newspaper wrote an article about Catherine and we collected $1600 in pledges for our family to complete the five mile walk. We had a great time walking and enjoyed spending the day with the clinic staff in such an informal environment. Formal Dr. Truman completed the walk in his suit and tie, which Catherine thought was hysterical. She was also delighted that one of her classmates made the walk with her. We passed through the fall months happily enough and celebrated Thanksgiving with my sister and her family in California, taking in Disneyland and celebrating the end of treatment which was coming. We felt tremendous relief that we had defeated leukemia and that Catherine would soon be done with her struggle.

In the treatment summary dated November 30, 1983 in Catherine's medical records, it says *discontinue chemo;* just an inch away from those words in bold red lettering are the words *CYTOLOGY POSITIVE.*

From the Journal, December 3, 1983:

Catherine has relapsed. There are no words to describe the horror, the pain, the fear and the incredible nightmare through which we are living. It is a Central Nervous System Relapse. To save her, the strongest measures are needed. To start, there will be three spinal taps per week for as long as it takes to bring things under control, after that one spinal per week for six months and then one per month after that. That alone should be enough, but on top of it comes cranial and spinal radiation—also assorted vincristine and prednisone doses and who knows what else—cytosine, CCNU, cytoxan, 6-thioguanine, asparaginase, adriamycin, hydrocortisone, methotrexate. We can do it, but the catch to the whole thing is it might not work. The uncertainty is horrible. Catherine is frightened and suffering, but she is also strong and brave. Matthew is tired of the whole business. We are all in shock and the fear will have to settle down or we can't go on.

21

Settling Down

At the clinic the next day, every diagnostic test available was run. Everyone clung to the slim hope that a laboratory mistake had been made, yet everyone knew it was highly unlikely. The pathology report indicated 352 leukemia cells per milliliter of fluid on November 30 and the next test run only two days later showed 906. There was no doubt. The good news for us that day was that there seemed to be no bone marrow involvement, with cells found only in the central nervous system. With Catherine still lying on the exam table waiting for the final news, I stepped out into the hallway with Dr. Truman and asked him how we could possibly do it all again. He said, *The person who will show you the way is sitting right in there waiting for us.* He was upset himself, but he was correct in his assessment of from where the strength would come.

We began the new protocol that morning in the clinic. The diagnostic spinal tap needle, left in place in her spine while we waited for the analysis to confirm the relapse, became the conduit for the first of many doses of methotrexate injected directly into the spinal fluid. The effectiveness of the treatment was clear to us; after one dose of chemotherapy, the number of leukemia cells in the fluid sample of December 5 was down to 68 per milliliter. We prepared ourselves to face the new three year protocol designed to reduce the number to 0.

After the new protocol was begun we simply went home. Catherine wanted to go to school so I took her. We talked to her teacher, who as a former nurse fully understood the impact of the relapse. She affectionately put Catherine to work with her group and assured me in the hallway outside the classroom that she would do her part. I knew she could be counted on. As I walked down the

Cynthia Krumme

long school hall, our friend Paul with whom we had celebrated just two nights before appeared. I told him what had happened and I cried on his shoulder as he held me up with his assurances that we were not alone. Catherine made it through the rest of the day, supportively distracted by her second grade class. I went home and started making the phone calls to tell our families that we must begin again.

From the medical records, December 5, 1983:

> *Catherine had a good weekend. She feels relatively well. Jaw pain and a "sore mouth." Sue Thompson, RN.*

From the Journal, December 7, 1983:

> *Catherine was a "warrior" at the clinic today. She was powerful. Her goal was to overcome fear and pain and she did it. The fear of the spinals is the real problem, she can handle the pain. Today she showed her power over the fear.*

By December 9, Catherine was in remission. The cell count was only 2 per milliliter of fluid, near the threshold of detection, and the decision was made to cut down to one spinal per week. We were given the maintenance schedule which we found to be incredibly aggressive. Already she was having difficulty keeping food in her stomach and she had to drag herself through the school day. She was humiliated that week when she threw up in school. For weeks she felt nauseated and broke out in hives every day. Just as she had done for three years, she went to school every day except when she had to be at the clinic. She considered it her job to go and she benefited from the support of her thoughtful teacher and from the presence of her classmates. The school principal was not convinced that it was good for Catherine to be in school, but she accepted our decision.

From Catherine's pre-relapse story, October 5, 1983:

> *Last year in music class I felt sick one day. I bent over because that was the only way that I felt good. The music teacher said stand up we are about to do a dance. I think it was my medicine that made me feel bad. Finally I went to the school nurse and my mom came to pick me up there. That was the only time I felt sick in school, although sometimes I feel sick in the morning and don't want to go to school. But*

I go anyway because my mom says that I should try to tough it out. I usually feel much better when I get near my friends. Sometimes I get headaches in school, but I don't count that as being sick.

Catherine was in the clinic so much that she had the opportunity to develop a fast friendship with Lauren whom we had seen on TV and who had also had a relapse. The two girls and their nurse Sue spent hours together deep in conversations of all kind. Facing innumerable spinal taps, Catherine worked out her own position for the procedure, wherein she sat tailor fashion bent over a pillow which had the effect of rounding off her spine. The staff let her have her own way about this and she seemed to handle the LPs better.

From the Journal, December 11, 1983:

Dr Truman has urged me to write down what he calls "Catherineisms." While chatting away with each other during the waiting period of a spinal tap, Catherine looked over her shoulder at Dr. Truman and said, "Having leukemia isn't so bad. Of course it wouldn't be my first choice."

During these early days of the relapse, Catherine and I were asked to schedule one of her visits during a time when the MGH Board of Trustees would be touring the clinic. Dr. Truman asked Catherine to explain to the Board what it was like to get a spinal tap and frequent IVs.

From the Journal, December 17, 1983:

She said that the spinal hurts a lot for one minute and then the other nine minutes are not much. She told them about her breathing and how it helps her and she said that she likes to chat with Dr. Truman and her parents during the spinals. With regard to the IVs, she said there is nothing to them. Once you've had a spinal, an IV is nothing. She looked beautiful sitting there on the bed telling them about her illness. Dr. Truman said that we all thought we had beaten Catherine's leukemia, but we were wrong, so we are going to beat it this time. I think he is right.

Most of December was spent in the clinic. Matt came with us

when he could and we were surrounded by supportive parents and friends there. Catherine enjoyed getting to reach into the toy box at every visit and we made some trips on our own to purchase special toys that she would enjoy finding there. She and Lauren planned for Christmas and we became friends with her parents. David became a regular blood donor that Christmas because Lauren needed blood transfusions. Because we were at the clinic so often, we came into frequent contact with other children who had suffered a relapse. Those children were fighting with all their strength to survive, and they were determined to enjoy life. Knowing the clinic families was a profoundly moving part of the cancer treatment.

From Catherine's second grade paper, December 12, 1983:

Dear Santa, I have been a good girl this year. I would like an orange in my stocking and maybe some make-up. If you could, I would like you to make my leukemia go away soon. Love, Catherine.

Christmas was wonderful that year. People shopped for us, baked the cookies that we didn't have time to bake, and offered any support they could. Word of the relapse spread like wildfire. Friends responded with offers of help and letters poured in. Someone found the special doll that Catherine had wanted that was already sold out in the stores; the cookies and fixings for gingerbread houses were delivered one pre-Christmas day; and Matthew lit a "candle of caring" in his Sunday School chapel and dedicated it to his sister. We didn't know what to say, it was all so overwhelming. We did our best to take part in our normal holiday activities. Catherine and Matthew sang in their school holiday program, we went to the committee meetings that we normally attended, we went to a party, David's parents came for New Year's and we celebrated being together. We knew that Catherine would lose her long hair soon from the intense chemotherapy, so on the day after Christmas we went to a wig specialty store and matched her hair color on a wig she liked. The people at the store were helpful and considerate. Within a week after the wig purchase all of Catherine's hair fell out. Matthew worried that he would not like to see her without hair, but of all of us he was the most supportive, telling her daily how pretty she was. He rose to the occasion just as he had since the beginning. We prepared for the children to return to school and we settled down to the business at hand.

Letter from Robert Storer, retired Unitarian minister, December, 1983:

Dear Catherine, Just a line from Texas to tell you I am thinking of you and I hope and pray that your treatment is helping. Keep up your fine spirit.

Catherine's January, 1984 letter to her Icelandic friend:

Dear Helga, The medicine I take for leukemia has made my hair fall out. I have much less hair than I had in kindergarten. I'm also sick in bed with the flu. I'm not sure if I will be able to come visit you until my leukemia is gone. Love, Catherine

January, 1984 letter to my parents:

Matthew has been a great help to Catherine throughout this whole ordeal. She has now lost every bit of her hair. He pats her on the head and tells her that her head has a nice shape and he likes it. We bought her a wig which she wears to school sometimes, although it is cute, she doesn't like it much. She prefers to wear a brightly colored scarf in turban fashion. She looks darling.

January, 1984 letter to a California friend whose own child died of leukemia years before:

Oh my perceptive friend, how I wish I did not have to write this letter to you or anyone else, but the time has come. No Christmas letter this year because Catherine's leukemia has relapsed and I didn't want to fill a Christmas letter with such news. The relapse is in the Central Nervous System and was discovered in the final spinal tap that is done when one goes off treatment. We went home to celebrate and received a call the next day that the pathologists had found a few suspicious cells in her spinal fluid. A CNS relapse is the best kind one can have, but it is definitely a major setback for her and for us all. We have begun the entire chemotherapy experience over again and happily she is already in remission again. The chemo will be much more aggressive this time and we are all gearing up for a long siege. We believe with gut-level surety that she will make it. She is handling the experience very well as is Matthew. Both children started out angry and now are all ready to do battle. Matthew said the first time was a battle like "Star Wars" and then "The Empire Struck Back," but now it's time for "The Return of the Jedi!" I thought it was an apt analogy. David and I are taking a lot of courage from our lovely children. Other than that shocking ending, we had a great year. We think we have managed to retain our sense of humor, but at the least we have pulled ourselves together. Try not to worry, just hold us in your heart as we do you.

22

New Treatments

In January of 1984 we began the complicated maintenance therapy. The program consisted of an eight week cycle with a different combination of drugs given every two weeks. Each combination was designed to attack the remaining cancer cells in a different way, on the theory that cells that might be resistant to one kind of attack might be vulnerable to another. Each drug had a specific function and each drug carried with it the possibility of any number of strange side effects. It is the appropriate policy of medical treatment today to inform the patients and their families of the risks of treatment, so we were given information sheets for each drug which detailed all possible side effects, from the common to the bizarre. Among the possibilities were hair loss, weight loss, weight gain, nausea and vomiting, bone marrow depression, liver changes, constipation, numbness, tingling, hand tremors, muscle cramps, weakness of arms or legs, pain in the jaw, heart changes, mouth sores, lower abdominal pain, stomach irritation, diarrhea, fever, phlebitis, increased appetite, high blood pressure, stomach irritation, sensitivity to the sun, puffiness in cheeks, nightmares, diabetes, bleeding in the bladder, and sterility, to name a few. We knew from experience not to take the risks too seriously, but rather to be aware of them and to be cautious about following all diagnostic and prophylactic measures that were recommended. I'm sure that in those days Catherine drank more water than any child her age because I was convinced it would flush her system!

Since Catherine would be receiving adriamycin, which may over time affect the heart, it was necessary to record a base line echocardiogram before her first dose. It could be compared with others

---

taken every few months to monitor any changes in heart size, beat strength, or valve operation that might be caused by adriamycin. Catherine did not like participating in the echocardiogram then or any other time. She said the pressure on her chest for the lengthy time it took to get a reading was too much. She complained more about this test than the spinals, even though it was a non-invasive test.

In the car on the way to the clinic one cold January day, Catherine made up a list of rules she thought should be followed if one were to have a successful children's cancer clinic. She presented the rules to her doctor. The Clinic Rules still hang on the wall, just as true today as they were then.

Clinic Rules

1. *Must have a good sense of humor.*
2. *Must always do a good LP and Bone Marrow.*
3. *Must always remember the toy box.*
4. *Must tell the truth.*
5. *Must like people.*
6. *Must like junk food.*
7. *Must know a lot about chemotherapy.*
8. *Must not mind the sight of blood.*
9. *Must like bald heads.*
10. *Must never be grumpy.*

The first two-week cycle was thioguanine and cytoxan; the second, adriamycin; the third, methotrexate and CCNU ("the bomb"); and fourth, vincristine, dexamethazone and cytosine arabinoside. We followed this routine for three years, interrupted only by low counts which prevented chemo occasionally, and by some mixing up of the schedule to allow for the drugs she tolerated best to be given just before vacations or other important occasions. The ability and willingness of the doctors to adapt the rigid schedule to our needs reflected a human touch that made a big difference for us and the other families.

The clinic staff tried to keep the waiting at a minimum, but it was not always possible. Emergencies always took precedence of course, but human needs also took extra time. We never went to the clinic and left feeling that we didn't have time to talk about our concerns. This courtesy was policy and while we did our share of waiting for others to finish, we benefited from the attention when our turn came. Waiting is part of the cancer experience and we became experts at it.

From the Journal, January 12, 1984:

We spent six hours at the clinic today, much of it waiting for treatment to begin. Catherine was scared during the spinal, but rallied when it was over. The cytoxan is adminis- tered in an IV solution and dripped in with large amounts of fluid to prevent dehydration. It took two hours and wore us out. By the time we got home with Matthew and some McDonald's hamburgers, it was 7 p.m. Another long day.

During this period, a CAT scan was scheduled for Catherine, both to establish a base line and to see if there was any tumor evidence. This particular diagnostic procedure was a most unpleas- ant experience. We did not understand that there would be an additional IV administered and we did not prepare our daughter for one in advance as we always tried to do. We had the custom of always being with her during these times, but due to the nature of the test we were not permitted in the room. Had I known there was to be an IV, I would have insisted on being with her while it was inserted and then leave. We were surprised that the supervising doctor never came out of the closed room to meet us or to tell us any information either before or after the test. We were angered and defensive about not being included in the distribution of information, and we were upset that our child was left alone in a situation in which she might have needed support. To complicate the situation, we were told by a technician who brought Catherine out of the room that things looked *odd*. He asked us, *Does she have a history of hygroma?* but then would not tell us what that was. Our dictionary described hygroma as, in essence, water on the brain. It was Saturday and we brooded for the rest of the weekend. Happily, on Monday at the clinic Dr. Truman said the CAT scan was perfectly normal. With a mixture of annoyance and mirth, he rejected the red herring in one word: *Hygroma!* Catherine commented that she figured out when they started to talk about an IV on Saturday that no one had told her mom in advance, otherwise she'd be there. She assured us she had handled it just fine!

At the end of January, the chicken pox immunity that had been achieved from the vaccination seemed to disappear. The doctor in charge of the immunization study felt it was possible that the heavy induction therapy required to achieve a remission was masking the titer. We were disappointed.

From a letter to my parents, January 21, 1984:

> *Some of the drugs make Catherine uncomfortable but the effects do not last long. At the same time that we are getting all this new treatment, many diagnostic tests have been ordered to establish a base line of all of Catherine's normal functioning so that the drug doses can effectively be altered to reduce long term side effects. She has had an echocardiogram, EKG, and today she goes in for a CAT scan. Once she found out that her grandad had had one and so had some of her clinic friends, she is actually looking forward to it. She is tremendously resilient. There is still no decision as to when the radiation will be given.*

Just as in the past, Catherine developed mouth sores from methotrexate, but on the new protocol the sores happened with every dose and they sometimes made eating impossible. She lost weight and strength. We could see by mid February that life was going to be more difficult, and David and I spent hours of our time together trying to figure out how to deal with each event. We literally talked our way through the relapse. Dr. Truman consulted colleagues around the country about their experiences with CNS relapse.

From the medical record, February 16, 1984:

> *Good month! No problems at all. (CAT scan neg.) Begin MTX-CCNU. Collecting opinions re cranial RT vrs cranio-spinal RT. J. Truman.*

From a letter to Dr. Keefer, HCHP, from Dr. Truman, February 21, 1984:

Thank you for your note. I'm embarrassed not to find any follow-up letter to you. I guess I'm just as possessive as a grandfather about my leukemia patients, especially the pretty ones, and sometimes I forget that anyone else is seeing them at the same time.

As you know, Catherine completed her 3 years of standard chemotherapy on 11-30-83, at which time, much to our dismay, we found that she had asymtomatic leukemic meningitis. She responded wonderfully to intrathecal chemotherapy on December 2, 5, and 7 and by December 9 had no further visible cells. She continued on weekly intrathecal treatment for six weeks, and has just graduated to monthly injections for the rest of the year (until Nov.). However, her systemic chemotherapy becomes more complex as the enclosed protocol indicates. She will be getting 8 drugs given via 2-week cycles, all of which are tolerated remarkably well. Indeed Catherine continues as the picture of good health. The only decision remaining is whether to give her cranial radiation therapy or cranial plus spinal radiation. I am in touch with my colleagues around the country about this, and I will soon have a consensus of opinion. I will give you a call about this.

Thank you for your continuing support. I am still very optimistic that cure is obtainable. With best wishes.

On February 28, 1984, Catherine got the pump for the first time. Wearing the infusion pump, which would deliver a continuous dose of cytosine over a 24-hour period, would require insertion of a butterfly IV needle in her skin at stomach level. Catherine would then connect the pump to the butterfly tubing and attach it by velcro to her strawberry decorated belt. Sue held out her arm to me, handed me the small IV needle, and said, *Practice here.* After successfully inserting the needle under the skin of her forearm, I turned and inserted a needle in the tummy of my daughter, just as I would do scores of times in the future. It felt like pushing a needle through layers of textured cloth, and then it was done. It was a hard day. Over the years, the pump was always difficult, both because of the insertion and because of the impact of the cytosine arabinoside, but Catherine and I talked it through many times and we both completely understood why it was so important.

From the Journal, March 1, 1984:

> *I put the sub-cutaneous needle in yesterday and again today and I'll do it again tomorrow. It is very difficult, but we are both OK. Catherine is upset and frightened, but is brave, in spite of not feeling well at all. Catherine broke down today and cried over her relapse. She said she wanted to be normal by now—she had planned on it and she wanted to be. I told her she is normal to us. It was heartbreaking to hear her cry, but I think she needed to and it has helped clear the air. She went to bed early and fell softly asleep.*

The highlight for Catherine at the clinic that winter was her growing friendship with twelve-year-old Lauren, whom she idolized. They commiserated, laughed, played jokes on Sue, on each other, and on their parents, and generally kept everyone's spirits up. They enjoyed going places together and including Sue and her boyfriend in their outings. Catherine's illness matured her in some ways, and as Lauren became more sick she enjoyed our daughter's company immensely. The age difference between the girls did not matter to them at all.

The new protocol was complicated to remember in the context of a busy life and we worried about making errors regarding taking the correct type or number of pills. We devised a series of symbols which I wrote on the kitchen calendar weekly and checked off when the medication had been given. Catherine would help by checking each day to be sure we had a mark though the medication symbol. Each family we knew devised their own plan for dealing with their part of the protocol, and for the most part people seemed successful with that aspect of the treatment. One day when were were discussing what to do because Catherine had vomited her medication within a minute of swallowing it and we were concerned about the loss of effectiveness, Sue told us a "clinic story." There was a family whose little son had had a great deal of difficulty swallowing his pills. The mother had tried many ways to give the medication and had finally hit on a successful method which she told one day in the clinic as their three year protocol was ending. She simply placed his methotrexate tablets on frozen pizza, baked them in the oven, and he ate them right up. Everyone was horrified, as cooking the medication could reduce or ruin its potency, but the child survived. Sue said, *Well, it seems to have worked!* Catherine loved the story and joked about it for years afterward.

Toward the end of March 1984, we began to prepare for cranio-spinal radiation therapy. Catherine was eager to get it over with.

Radiation Therapy

In late March, we first met with Dr. Linggood, the radiologist who would be handling Catherine's case. Dr. Truman, in his telephone inquiries around the country, got unpublished results from St. Jude's which seemed promising. Both Dr. Truman and Dr. Linggood recommended full cranial radiation plus spinal radiation, a procedure that was showing increased protection against bone marrow relapse in cases like Catherine's. For myself, once I had accepted that radiation was necessary, it seemed reasonable to use the form of radiation that would protect her to the fullest. The radiologist explained that fourteen courses of radiation would be applied over a two and a half week period. It amused us that we were to be given weekends off! She designed a set of radiation blocks to fit Catherine's body to protect her from receiving radiation in areas other than the ones targeted. We all appreciated the good natured approach of the Radiology Department and consequently entered into the treatment with an upbeat attitude. The week before we began, a late winter storm took out our power lines and it was 60 hours before the power returned. We spent those days trying to keep the house warm enough to prevent the pipes from freezing. Matthew began a research report on leukemia for his fourth grade teacher.

The logistics of going daily to the hospital presented some difficulties. Our friend Susan volunteered to drive. We took her up on her offer several times when David couldn't leave his classes. Judy and Paul kept Matthew after school on some days and on others he came with us to offer moral support for Catherine.

From the Journal, April 4, 1984:

Radiation Day Three. We are doing fairly well—no major side effects—in fact, tonight Catherine is quite chipper. They have had quite a bit of trouble with the "blocks" but seem to have straightened it out now. Dr. Linggood tells us she is very picky about getting the eyes properly protected. We appreciate her caution. At best I will never love radiation, but I'm trying not to hate it! Catherine, of course, is wonderful.

Matthew joined us for the next few days and interviewed the technicians for his leukemia report. From *Leukemia*, a report by Matthew Krumme, age 10, April 27, 1984:

Radiation is used to kill blasts. It is very effective, and it kills blasts by the thousands. Radiation is used in the head (Doctors call the head a cranium) and the spinal cord. Radiation comes out of a big machine. It will travel right through the air and into the body. It makes the hair fall out. This is because when the radiation is looking for blasts, it will look in the holes where the hair grows. The radiation will push the hair out.

To get the radiation in the right places, they will have to draw marks on the cranium and spinal cord. That way the radiation will get in only the places where it is needed. If it got in the eyes, it might make the patient blind. The doctors would always measure the cranium and the back to make sure everything would go right.

Each day of radiation, Catherine's blood counts were evaluated and the information was used to decide how much radiation would be appropriate on that day. Catherine would enter the room, lie down on the radiation bunk, and lie absolutely still for the ten minutes required for the dose to be set up and administered. We were required to wait behind a barrier in the outside hallway just behind the nurses station, where we could see her over closed circuit TV. She could hear our voices over the loudspeaker. While it was difficult to watch, we felt connected to her over the TV. She handled these procedures as if there was nothing to them. After four days of radiation, Catherine did not have a single hair on her head. She reported every day and still remembers vividly that the radiation had a distinctive, unpleasant odor that she found annoying. Sometimes when riding home in the car she would be nauseated so we carried a bowl with us just in case. Susan and I discovered that if Catherine was granted her wish to ride in the backward-facing seat of the station wagon, she would definitely need to use the bowl.

From the medical record, April, 1984:

The treatments were well tolerated and Catherine was an extremely cooperative and particularly nice child. 13 fractions over 17 elapsed days: brain; 13 fractions over 17 elapsed days: spine. Dr. Rita Linggood.

From the Journal, April 19, 1984:

Radiation over! Catherine appears to be fine. She is her old self. Thank goodness. We celebrated at a restaurant for dinner. The radio-tech gave her a chocolate bunny, a certificate of graduation, and a set of lavender barrettes for her wig. I hope it worked. We are feeling a bit desperate.

Generally speaking, the radiation treatment passed smoothly. Catherine continued to see Lauren in their free time and it became increasingly clear to her that Lauren was not likely to survive.

From Matthew's school report, April 27, 1984:

My sister has leukemia, but she is very brave. In fact, I don't think there are too many people who cooperate as well as she does. To live with a brother or sister with leukemia isn't hard if you know what to do. They are on treatment. It might mean he or she gets crabby, but you just don't say anything. When he or she is cheerful, be cheerful with them. If you ever get jealous, just tell your parents. In many cases, leukemia is a treatable disease. People who have it can look forward to healthy happy lives.

From January of 1984 to the summer of 1985, Catherine had either no hair or almost no hair. For the most part this did not bother her, although she did have some problems with one class-mate who teased her about wearing a wig. We approached the teacher for help and ended up with Catherine initiating a discussion with the girl and telling her a bit about what she was experiencing. While the girls did not become best friends, the teasing about hair ceased. She wore the wig to school and discarded it the minute she got home, usually by pulling it off at the kitchen door and letting it fly across to the counter top where it would land in a heap. Her friends accepted her completely. One afternoon at gymnastics, the wig slipped during a somersault. Catherine was embarrassed by this, even though she realized the other children didn't notice. As time went on, she developed a certain bravado about having no hair, and outside of school she would wear her wig or not depending on whether it was hot or cold.

From 15-year-old Catherine, November 1991:

Losing my hair didn't seem to bother me that much. I remember going over to a friend's house and popping off my wig whenever it got too hot. I never did that in school, but my friends didn't seem to mind.

24

I Want to Have Hot Chocolate on the Champs Élysées

Our family loved to travel, and in spite of leukemia, Catherine had grand aspirations and a great deal of interest in travel, too. We had taken several trips, but had not been back to Europe since her diagnosis, largely because we were concerned about carrying her medication with us and getting help for her if it was needed. We had traveled in the United States and had always said we would see Europe again when Catherine was through with her treatment. The reality of the relapse caused us to rethink this position and we decided to take a family trip to Paris at a time when the foreign exchange rate was favorable. Ever since she was little, Catherine had said she wanted to have hot chocolate on the Champs Élysées and we decided to make her dream come true in late May, 1984.

As we finished up radiation and began to plan for our trip in earnest, we took time to see Lauren and her family and enjoyed a memorable trip to our local fair with them. Lauren's father, Bob, played the arcade games and won several stuffed dolls for both girls. The day was warm and so was the company.

From Catherine's second grade paper, May 21, 1984:

The Enka Fair came to Winchester and I rode almost everything. My favorite ride was the Super Slide. I went on that twice. I also like the Sizzler. My wig almost blew off on the rides. I had loads and loads of fun.

From a letter from Lauren's mother Louise, May 1984:

We enjoyed seeing your home and enjoyed Winchester. We thank you for a wonderful day at the fair on Saturday. It was just great for us and hope it was the same for you. Have a safe trip to Paris. Be sure to remember us to Dr. Robbins. She is one of our favorite people. We look forward to spending a day with you when you return.

The week before our departure for Paris, Catherine was given adriamycin. The medication schedule was altered so she would not have to wear the pump in France. A friend called to tell me how worried she was about Catherine, having seen her and observing that she seemed disoriented and weak. The medication frequently took its toll. Rarely did people comment on Catherine's appearance. Sometimes when she looked the most ill she was actually doing very well, and we frequently told people that her appearance did not necessarily correlate with her well being. Notably, when the relapse occurred, she looked terrific, pink cheeked and robust. We knew that looks weren't everything.

Dr. Robbins, a former clinic fellow, was working in Paris for a few years. At the suggestion of Dr. Truman, we wrote to her expressing our interest in saying hello when we arrived. She was a very popular person at the clinic so we were delighted to carry everyone's good wishes to her. In addition, knowing she was there gave us a connection to the clinic just in case we needed any help while in Europe. The trip was wonderful. We invited David's parents along and the six of us stayed in a hotel owned by the parents of one of David's students at Tufts. They treated us as special guests. We met Dr. Robbins for tea and she introduced us to the best macaroons in Paris. While in Paris, we went to the opera and sat in a red velvet-lined box seat, we toured the museums, we shopped, we rode the subway and the buses, and we had hot chocolate on the Champs Élysées. David and I celebrated our 15th wedding anniversary, convinced that we would make everyone's life the best we could. In the pictures of that trip, we all look thin and tired with big smiles on our faces. Smiling Catherine, who always looked great to us, appears frail in those photos.

We returned home renewed and carrying special little gifts for special clinic friends. Catherine picked out French perfume in a lovely cut glass bottle for Lauren. By now Catherine clearly understood that Lauren had only a short time left and she wanted to share Paris with her. We went to Lauren's home for a special party a week after we returned home. Lauren made Catherine a lavender and pink bead bracelet and the girls floated on air mattresses in Lauren's pool, while Catherine chattered away about the trip. Lauren was subdued and when we left she hugged Catherine and said she hoped to see her again soon. The next week when we saw Lauren in the clinic, she was very ill. That was the last time the girls saw each other and Lauren was so weak that Catherine did all the hugging. Catherine slept through most of the two weeks after that, a delayed result of the radiation therapy. The period of radiation sleep was distressing. Catherine rarely left her bed even to eat and it was just too much like losing her.

From the medical record, June, 1984:

> *Catherine is feeling well. No problems. She has been very tired—probably "sleepy time" due to radiation. Sue Thompson, RN.*

Lauren Marie Belyea died on July 12, 1984. Two other teenagers from our clinic died in the same month. The losses turned the clinic upside down emotionally and it took the rest of the summer for the tension there and at home to ease up. The devoted clinic secretary decided to leave the front lines and work on the statistics in the back office, and by fall, dear Sue had decided to work only part time. We were reminded of the terrible strain that the clinic personnel work under. The losses hurt us deeply, but we did not live them every day as these devoted people did. We did however, have a child with the same disease, and during that summer we sometimes felt that we were riding a derailed train.

On June 15, 1988, Catherine wrote:

Lauren, A True Friend

Since when does red hair and freckles allow you to make

other people crack up all the time? I've never met such a joker as twelve-year-old Lauren. I've never met such a good friend as Lauren either. She was always so happy and when the going got tough she always lifted my seven-year-old spirits. You see we both had one major thing in common. We both had a blood disease called leukemia.

You might say that leukemia was our shared problem at that time and she always made me feel like we really were going to beat it. When I was with her, I never thought about the bad times. When someone jokes about every other medicine you're taking you forget about how things hurt! At least I did. Lauren made me feel that way. She was my true friend and even though I only knew her less than a year, she was my best friend.

Lauren, our nurse Sue, and I made quite a trio. Even though Lauren was quite a trooper, she never liked getting anything done to her. She didn't like IVs, she didn't like pills or anything of the sort, and sometimes she used to try to avoid getting something. I remember her saying, "You know Sue, I don't think we have to do this today," or, "Do you really think this is necessary?" Of course the answer would always be yes.

I always thought it was ironic how Lauren always made me feel confident about my illness, but she was not so confident about hers. Just before my eighth birthday, Lauren died. A couple of months before this, when she knew she was going to die, she just wasn't her spunky self and as much as I loved her I wanted her to be the way she was. I miss her so much that I usually forget about the end because Lauren, in my opinion, was the greatest!

From Matt's college essay, Fall, 1991:

When I was eleven and Catherine was almost eight, a girl named Lauren died of leukemia. Lauren had been my sister's best friend and the pain for her at that time was probably worse than any pain she had ever felt from her chemo-therapy. Lauren's funeral was the first I had ever been to.

Catherine had been referred to an ophthalmologist to have her eyes checked. The appointment, for which we had waited over a month, fell on the morning of Lauren's funeral. We planned to go to the appointment, eat lunch afterwards, and then drive directly to the funeral location on the south shore, a distance of about 30 miles. The visit to the eye doctor went badly. We were already saddened by losing Lauren and I explained to the doctor that we had a time constraint because we were going to her funeral. The ophthalmologist kept us waiting for over an hour and a half in spite of my plea. Finally he called Catherine in, spent five minutes with her, and abruptly told her she would have to wear glasses. When I responded with an involuntary, *Oh no,* he criticized me for not accepting the idea of wearing glasses, an interesting concept because I have worn them myself for nearly 30 years. We left the office, prescription in hand, determined never to see that doctor again, and drove, without time for lunch, to arrive just as the service began. Later at the graveside, Louise and Bob stopped talking with others, came over to Catherine and told her how much they loved her. They warmly greeted Matthew and tried to cheer us up when they were the ones who had lost their daughter. We had come to be with them and there they were comforting us. They demonstrate the best in people.

Letter from Lauren's mother, August 3, 1984:

Dear loving friends, It is impossible to express in words our thanks to you for all the love and support you have given us during these difficult months. Lauren truly loved you as we do. You were a very bright part of her life and she did enjoy doing things with Catherine so much. Thank you also for your gift in Lauren's memory to Mass. General. Their loving care to our children is really a gift to all of us and I'm so pleased that so many people have expressed their sympathy by sending gifts there. You are in our thoughts and prayers. God bless you. Our little girls are so very precious and special. Love, Louise

In the summer of 1984, Dr. William Ferguson joined the clinic as a clinical and research fellow. Based on his accomplishments we expected a stuffy fellow, but what we got was a warm funny fellow who won our hearts. The first time we met him, Catherine was due to receive vincristine and in walked Dr. Ferguson holding a tray of medication with an above-the-head flourish, like a waiter who is serving royalty. He announced with great decorum, *Coffee, tea, or vincristine?* Catherine had the best doctors we have ever met.

On August 3, Catherine celebrated her eighth birthday with a sleep over party that she hosted with her bald head decorated with stick-on ribbons. The morning of her party, David and I attended the funeral of an 18-year-old clinic friend who died of a brain tumor. In the afternoon we served cake to ten laughing, lively little girls. Our lives were full of stark contrasts. The grief of the summer of 1984 wore us all down.

In September, Catherine headed back to school wearing her new adorable red glasses and her wig. My mother, who had become bedridden with osteoporosis, went to stay temporarily in California with my sister where she could get regular therapy. Feeling lonely, my father came to see us and spent his time cheering up the children. This visit was the first time any of our parents had seen Catherine when she was having significant difficulties. Dad was very supportive and his visit cheered us. He watched the children's soccer games, took them to McDonald's, teased and cajoled Catherine into eating when she had little appetite, and encouraged us to plan another "mental health" trip, this time to London, which we planned for the day after Christmas. We felt back on track.

From the medical records, September 17, 1984:

> *Catherine experienced back pain for two days following her last vincristine injection. She also complained of joint pain in arms, legs and abdominal area. Otherwise she is doing very well. Sue Thompson, RN.*

From a letter to friends in Washington, November, 1984:

> *Dear friends, try not to worry too much when you don't hear from us . . . it has more to do with being busy and having time just slip away than anything else. Please know that I will let you know right off if we need something or if things change here. One of the big problems of living with*

a serious illness is that it is very tiring both emotionally and physically for all members of the family. We spend about one full day a week in the clinic with Catherine and that's a lot of time spent in that environment. In the last year alone, we have lost 17 friends to cancer. Over the summer, Catherine's best friend from the clinic died and we have mourned her greatly. Sometimes we wonder how much more Catherine can stand or Matthew can stand or we can stand, but most of the time we feel strong and united and in fact happy with each other and with our lives. We are certainly happy with our friends and the longtime support they have offered us. We love you.

25

I've Been Having a Wonderful Life So Far

On the first day back at school that fall, I drove Catherine to school and went to see the school nurse with an update as was my habit. The school principal greeted me with the comment, *We are surprised to see Catherine back, she looked so bad last year we thought she wouldn't make it.* While I had come to expect certain responses in the school setting, I was completely at a loss for words. We had encouraged the principal to attend the clinic information meetings for school personnel and she had in fact done so; however, she remained unsensitized to the impact of her words. The school nurse stepped in to soothe the situation, and I filled her in on Catherine's medical condition and went home, stunned. We settled into the school routine. Catherine began to take the anti-nausea medication vistaril, with dramatic benefit. She was regaining her strength and doing well in school, but the many sadnesses of the clinic were hard on her. Fortunately, Catherine has always been able to express her feelings in a direct way. We usually know what is on her mind. When a two-year-old she knew died after a bone marrow relapse in October, she calmly observed to me that she had noticed that everyone with a bone marrow relapse died. She wondered aloud if she would have one. While she was very nearly correct in her assessment, as very few children survived except when the relapse was late or where marrow transplants were used successfully, she needed answers from us. We tried to help her understand and to give her the will to keep working hard at getting well.

Cynthia Krumme

From the Journal, October 17, 1984:

I told her that for her to spend her time worrying about a relapse was like worrying about falling off the porch and breaking a leg: it could happen, but time spent worrying about it doesn't help or make the event happen or not happen. It just makes you feel badly. She agreed, but wanted to know what would happen if she had a bone marrow relapse. I told her we would fight, not give up hope and make life the best we could, even if it wasn't for very long. I tried to reassure her that she is doing well even though it is hard for her. I asked her if she thought that Lauren had had a good life and she thought about it and said yes. She is a very thoughtful little girl. I feel proud of her and very sad that so much has happened to her in her short little life.

Throughout the fall Catherine had days when she felt well and days when the impact of chemotherapy was substantial. She went to school every day and we were able to work out a loose agreement with the teacher and the administrators that we would be allowed to make the judgement as to whether she should be in school. Prior to ironing this out, Catherine had frequently been told, by people who were moved to help her but who did not fully understand her situation, that she should stay home if she didn't feel well. If we had done this, Catherine might have missed school every day for three years. We discovered that the distraction and the companionship of classmates did a great deal to help her feel better. She found that putting her head down and resting for a short time often got her through the tough moments. A few times over the course of later treatment Catherine actually went to the nurse's office and lay down and was allowed to return to class at her own choosing. And occasionally, when a fever developed, she stayed home. However, during that third grade year it remained a struggle for us to convince the school that she should be there. In October, Catherine's teacher, the principal, and the school nurse attended the clinic's information session for educators. We hoped it would help them better appreciate Catherine's situation. At parent conferences in November, Matthew's teacher expressed his great interest in helping Matt and told us what a fine boy he was. Catherine's teacher expressed her concern that Catherine wasn't performing as she used to. The teacher seemed disappointed in her. She was unable to give us any examples of what she meant, but simply commented that Catherine seemed to be having difficulties. I felt awful after the conference, but I believed the teacher was having trouble accepting a child who might not survive. We knew that Catherine was a capable student and that she was the same as she had ever been, except for chemotherapy-induced fatigue. Catherine was happy in school and not aware of the teacher's feelings.

Catherine's school paper, December 14, 1984:

My name is Catherine Krumme and I discovered I had a disease called leukemia when I was four. I had to go to the hospital. When I came home my father built an above ground pool because I couldn't go to the public pool. I am now eight and enjoying school very much. Last summer I went to Paris, France. I am going to London for Christmas. I have been having a wonderful life so far.

26

A Tale from the Toy Box

The toy box in the clinic had long fascinated Catherine. When it was first placed there by the founders of the Charley Davidson Leukemia Fund, she rarely got to see inside it, but after the relapse she was eligible for a toy on almost every visit. She came away with crayons, books, small cars, a stuffed animal, and the occasional gift that we placed in there just for her. The toys were purchased by different people and an attempt was made to be sure that particular children got special wishes granted sometimes when they opened the box. Lauren was delighted one spring day to find a soft white stuffed seal which she had wanted. Once a big dump truck found its way into the box for an inquisitive four-year-old boy, and Top Forty cassette tapes and sophisticated books for certain teenagers appeared from time to time.

The toy box has a small padlock. Part of the thrill for the younger children is being able to track down the key and open it on their own. It sits in a corner of the treatment room and is used as a promise of pleasure to come for those who must endure another spinal, blood transfusion, or bone marrow test. Catherine unlocked that box scores of times and it helped her get through some tough times.

In December, we received a call from the den leader of the cub scout pack whose members came from Catherine's class. They wanted to take on the toy box as their Christmas project. To everyone's delight the project brought in about 50 small wrapped gifts each with a tag reflecting the age of the child for whom it would be appropriate. Catherine was thrilled when the huge stocking of gifts for the clinic arrived at our house. In what has since become a yearly ritual, we spread them out on the floor, checked to be sure they were tagged, added tape where necessary, and enjoyed the generosity of the scouts who had gathered them. We were delighted with the opportunity to play Santa at the clinic. That bag of gifts and the subsequent ones have brought big smiles to the faces of hundreds of children in the last decade. The tradition has continued despite several turnovers in the cub scouts and their adult leadership.

We celebrated Christmas with a vengeance. One year of relapse treatment down, two to go. Matthew had trouble sleeping and related, *I've never been in such a great Christmas spirit in my whole life.* On December 26th we left for 10 lovely days in London where we saw plays, museums, and tourist attractions until we had had our fill. We returned home, rested and eager to get on with life.

From the Journal, January 9, 1985:

> *Catherine had clinic on Monday—a spinal tap, vincristine, dexamethazone and the pump. The clinic was very hectic. Catherine is doing very well in spite of the difficult treatment. The school principal has taken a leave of absence and no one knows why.*

Two days later the school principal committed suicide. The school population reeled with the news and the remainder of the school year focused on understanding what had happened and putting in place a new principal. With the weight of this tragic occurrence, Catherine's illness was less of a concern to the interim administration and she just went about her business the best she could. Death was so much a part of our regular experience that we found we were not as shocked by this event as most of the school families were. We felt sorry for the loss of a life, but it was hard for us to reconcile an adult suicide when we watched young people who struggled so hard to live, and who sometimes died so painfully.

Cynthia Krumme

27

Muddling Through

The winter of 1985 brought more of the same. My mother was recovering from her back problems and had returned to her home in Louisiana much to everyone's delight. Our family pulled together to help the children accept the school tragedy. During that time David and I decided to begin to carve out some time for ourselves in which leukemia was not the only topic of conversation. We decided to plan a weekly dinner outing for ourselves and we did our best to set aside private time. The number of IVs that Catherine had over four years of chemotherapy began to take a toll on the small veins of her arms and hands.

From the Journal, February 4, 1985:

> *Adriamycin is getting harder and harder to deal with. Her veins won't cooperate and Sue wants to use veins in her feet. Catherine is terrified of the idea of needles in her feet. We will have to help her accept the idea if it would be better for her in the long run.*

In February of 1985, I gave the first of several talks to students in the local junior high. The curriculum called for discussion of important life events, and coping with critical or chronic illness was one of the events. I was initially uneasy about talking to students, but it proved a good experience for all concerned. I have repeated the talk to several classes over several years and have also spoken to school groups in other towns. In addition to these talks, we have all in various combinations spoken to groups ranging from nurses, doctors, students, parents, and patients.

In March, another of Catherine's clinic friends had a bone

---

marrow relapse. In early April, Catherine, Sue, and I spoke to student nurses at the Mass. General and at Holy Cross University. Catherine was and is wonderful in these talks. She told clinic stories and gave the students a real view of what living with cancer is like. The Holy Cross talk was given on an afternoon when she had had treatment in the morning and by the time it ended she was shaking and pale, but she wanted to finish speaking. She made a tremendous impression on the students. That same week, she complained of aches and pains we thought were due to a cold that kept her out of school. We took an extra trip into the clinic to check her blood counts as the family was planning a California trip to visit family in the next week. That clinic visit was a nightmare.

From the Journal, April 17, 1985:

Catherine's blood counts came back bad! The lab indicated that her white count was 34,000 and the doctor told us a bone marrow test needed to be done as a relapse was suspected. It was a horrible moment and I'm still having trouble with it. They were setting up the test tray when the lab called back to say there may have been a mistake—redraw the blood. Dr. Truman came running into the room to say, "Put your emotions on hold—there may have been a mistake." The clinic was in an uproar and very saddened at the prospect of a problem for Catherine. She was very fearful of the bone marrow test and not totally aware of the possibility of relapse or the potential that one would bring. I carried the blood to the lab myself, thinking if they see that she is a real girl with a real family maybe it will be all right. The lab had made an error. Catherine's count was 6,700. We all started to breathe again. Now that I know what it feels like, maybe we will be spared more knowledge.

From the medical records, April 12, 1985:

WBC initially reported as 34,000—severe concern re. bone marrow—machine error. John Truman.

This lab error is the only one I am aware of in our case in almost seven years of treatment. The shock of the event wore on us for weeks. To this day I vividly remember Monica coming into the room with Dr. Truman and putting her arm tightly around my shoulders, while Catherine sat straddle-legged on the exam table, and Dr. Truman saying, *The counts are bad.*

Our lives just rolled from one course of chemotherapy to the next. I wrote less in the journal that spring than any other time. The entries were full of pain. It wasn't that life was going so badly, it was just that it took all the energy we could muster to keep life normal. During this time, our small business began to flourish and I became a partner in a small video production company. Matthew began writing books and stories for everyone and played on a soccer team he loved and called "The Spoilers." Catherine played traveling team soccer for the first time and gave a party for her teammates at the end of the season. David finished up another year at Tufts and began his sabbatical year with great enthusiasm. Catherine continued to experience various side effects from her medications, in addition to the more serious ones associated with suppression of blood counts. She nearly always had back pain with vincristine, a rash after cytoxan in spite of the use of benadryl, and mouth sores from methotrexate. She coughed and had cold symptoms throughout her treatment.

From the medical records, June 10, 1985:

> *Catherine had a "bout" of mouth sores after methotrexate.*
> *Back pain severe, marrow suppression, future dose vincristine*
> *cut 50%. J. Truman.*

When school ended, we headed for our annual trip to Acadia National Park, which we hoped would provide some rest and quiet communing with nature. Catherine started the week with hives, an allergic response to cytoxan which passed, and she was able to swim, hike, and enjoy the beautiful weather. We were cautious to protect her and ourselves from sunburn which in her case could happen rather easily. At dinner on the anniversary night of Lauren's death, Catherine ordered fried clams explaining to us that Lauren had taught her to eat them on one of their many outings in Boston. We enjoyed the pleasant memory.

Back at home, the children went to soccer camp and settled in for some summer fun just lazing around. We received the news that my sister and her husband were separating as my brother and his wife had a few months before. The distance between our families made it difficult to do anything more than send love, but we suffered for them all. We would have liked to have helped them more. Catherine celebrated her ninth birthday on August 3rd. At the clinic that week we learned of the death of a thirteen-year-old and met old friends whose daughter had only a short time left. The hundreds of patients cured without relapse or other disaster always seemed to be overshadowed by the dozens for whom the treatment was less effective.

From the Journal, August 6, 1985:

We received jolting news at the clinic of a death and two relapses. Sue says the families are in bad shape. It was a terrible week for them.

The last week of August we set out for Colorado after enduring some ribbing from the clinic about our travel needs. We met wonderful people and had an excellent time. My sister and her son joined us as they would for the next several years.

Sabbatical

School started, fall soccer started, and David was in his home office doing independent research during his year-long sabbatical. With the children out of the house, we had some moments to talk alone and during that first week he told me he had wanted the sabbatical to occur during this year because he felt Catherine and the family needed him around more often. He was right. The new school principal called me for a meeting and indicated that it was her wish that Catherine be in school as much as possible and she would facilitate that in any way needed. School was easier for Catherine after her arrival.

Catherine loved her soccer team and in early September scored her first goal ever on a breakaway play from her position in the backfield. It was a moment of high drama and excitement. When we got home from the game she was running a fever and spent the next two days in bed. It was a weekend of contrasts, but we appreciated her determination to score that goal. She pushed herself as she did in everything. The strength of her will to be like everyone else was admirable. At the end of September, Hurricane Gloria swept through Massachusetts and took with it the top of our Norway Maple and our phone lines. We joked that it fit the uproar of our lives in general. In October, my parents visited, both in reasonably good health, and we had a fine visit. Matthew played pool with his grandfather and told me later he was glad he did. We felt the fall was going well for all of us.

From the Journal, November 8, 1985:

Jessica died yesterday. I told Catherine just now and she

is in her room "resting." We are all so saddened by Jess's death that we seem to be running in slow motion.

In late November, the chicken pox returned and we sent out the annual chicken pox letters again. Catherine was optimistic that she had a titer that was just being masked, and that everything would be fine. After the failure to register a titer in January, 1984, we could take no chances. However, her fourth grade class was spared and the design of the school allowed her to be segregated from the younger children where the disease was more prevalent. We spent Thanksgiving alone and invited David's parents and grandmother to visit at Christmas. Catherine was thrilled during the second week of December to be selected by tryout for the town-wide privately sponsored children's theater musical play, *Cinderella.* Just as in the schools and in sports, the environment surrounding the play was highly competitive. Being selected for this play at this time was a big boost to her emotional well-being. Catherine may well have been let into the Children's Theater group that first year because she tried so hard in the audition, looked so sick, and needed the group experience so much, but whatever the reason, she earned her position that year and in subsequent years through her hard work. The director of that theater was one of the few people we know of who ever gave Catherine a break because she was having a tough time. There may have been others who took her illness into consideration, but for the most part she lived her life by exactly the same rules as every other child her age in spite of her difficulties.

The toy box was once again filled by the scout troop and Matthew's sixth grade class raised $95 and purchased books and toys for older children. He felt proud. Christmas came and went and clinic visits continued to dominate our lives.

From the Journal, January 4, 1986:

Another New Year. 1985 was one of many changes, much happiness and much pain. Thank goodness we're all hanging in there.

From the Journal, January 26, 1986:

The time continues to move slowly by. Catherine is trying

very hard to keep going—so much time has passed and we have all lost so much. On Friday night, Catherine was away and Matthew was saying how much fun it was to have just the three of us at dinner, then suddenly he said, "But not all the time!" He can't imagine not having his sister with him. We were sobered by the thought and spent the rest of the meal trying to reassure him.

We rode an emotional roller coaster for years. Each one of us had moments where we let down and the others came forward with support. We were fortunate in that we were able to listen to each other and we didn't all fall apart at the same time!

With David on sabbatical, we decided to take advantage of the school's February vacation and head south for a peek at Williamsburg, Virginia. Leaving cold New England, we drove south to find temperatures in the 60s. We enjoy car trips and this one was special. On our second day in Williamsburg as we laughed and placed each other in the "stocks," we heard a woman's voice: *It's the Krummes!* We turned to see Lauren's parents, her older sister and her husband, and Lauren's little nephews running up to greet us. They lived about 30 miles from us and we had not seen them in a year, although we had spoken by phone and written. Like us, they had needed a break from winter and headed south.

From the Journal, February 23, 1986:

It was wonderful to see them. It is so hard to believe how much our lives are intertwined. Lauren was the focal point of our day with them, the glue that holds us together, and Catherine was the tangible evidence that life goes on. Bob hugged her with such longing and she responded with love. It was a high point.

All clinic parents expressed from time to time their fears about meeting up with families of the children that died. *What do you say? Will they resent the living? Will they survive emotionally? Will you be in their shoes someday? Are they too much of a tangible reminder of cancer?* Those questions always fade away when you stand with someone who has lived the same life, regardless of the outcome. Living with cancer is a bond that just glues people together. Most families who lose children are hungry for news of the other children. They want to know that their sacrifice may have made life better for someone else. They need to know what has become of the others. Many clinic families are tied together through success and through loss and they stand by each other.

We returned to Massachusetts refreshed. Business was brisk and we were devoting some energy to painting rooms in the house and repairing minor problems that had taken the back burner for years. Catherine was going daily to rehearsals for her play, and enjoying the freedom of acting, dancing, and singing. Her performance in March was wonderful. She had only a small part, but she played it for all it was worth. Her clinic friend Jason and his family came to the performance, much to her delight. Jason was recovering from a bone marrow transplant and we had great hopes for him.

We moved in on spring, judging time in terms of one course of treatment to the next, with a growing sense of confidence that we were winning the fight. The soccer season was a pleasant diversion, with David coaching both children's teams. Our dog Carter was showing signs of advanced age and we were aware that he didn't have much longer to live. My parents planned a move to a retirement community in San Antonio and eagerly looked forward to moving on May 5th.

From the medical record, May 12, 1986:

No problems at all. Playing forward on town soccer team. Now 2-1/2 years since resuming treatment. J. Truman.

From the medical record, May 27, 1986:

Catherine was not feeling well today. Attributes "blues" to many events. Not specific. Sue Thompson.

From the Journal, June 14, 1986:

My father, David O. Combs, died May 13, 1986 of a heart attack after one week in San Antonio. I am hurting.

We scattered my father's ashes off the Channel Islands in California. My mother decided to stay on in Texas and my sister and I worked out a program wherein we would each call her every other day for the foreseeable future. We loaded worry about her onto our already sagging shoulders.

From the Journal, June 25, 1986:

Our good old dog Carter died yesterday at age 15. Mom says Carter went to be with Dad. What a year.

It has never ceased to amaze us that at the same time cancer happens to a family, life in the outside world keeps happening at a frantic pace. One feels as if the world should stop and take notice, but it doesn't. Like all the clinic families we know, sorrow and joy hit us regularly and we just continued to put one foot in front of the other and go on—more or less.

The Last Six Months, Again

In June, Catherine's soccer team won first place in a local tournament, for which each girl won a trophy. We were thrilled for her because given the chemotherapy she had had the week before, we were somewhat surprised that she could run down the field at all. She had an enormous will to participate, and with the blessing of her doctors, she did. She looked triumphant on that field. We felt we needed to improve our spirits, and knowing my dad would have approved, we headed off to Bar Harbor to regroup. Once again we returned refreshed and with an improved outlook.

We had reached a state of mind where we were allowing ourselves to think about the end of treatment which we hoped would be in January 1987. Experience had shown us graphically that things can go wrong, but it is just not in our natures to expect the worst, so we expected the best and began to plan ahead. Adriamycin had been discontinued as a part of Catherine's protocol in late June due to evidence in her echocardiagram that her heart was being slightly adversely affected. This is a known side effect of the drug. There was a general feeling of relief at ending adriamycin as it frequently caused unpleasant side effects for her and because administration of the caustic drug in damaged veins was tricky and put everyone on edge. David liked to refer to adriamycin as equivalent to Drano. With the removal of adriamycin, the entire rotating protocol was moved from a two week cycle to a three week cycle. We noticed a certain optimism in the clinic personnel when they spoke of Catherine's future. We were buoyed up by all the changes.

From a letter to Dr. Keefer, HCHP, from Dr. Truman, July 22, 1986:

> *Just a brief note to let you know that Catherine Krumme has reached the 2-1/2 year point in her treatment for CNS recurrence. There have been no problems at all, though she has flirted with neutropenia on many occasions.*
>
> *She was due for her last dose of adriamycin today, but her echocardiagram showed slight decrease in left ventricular function relative to the prior echocardiagram; I hasten to add that her left ventricular function is still well within the normal range.*
>
> *I think we can now decrease the intensity of her chemo-therapy and move it to an every 3rd week cycle without adriamycin. Occasional surveillance LPs have been negative. Seeing that it is now over 5 years since she had leukemic cells in her bone marrow, I am increasingly optimistic that she will be cured. Very best wishes.*

David was enjoying his last months of sabbatical and was feeling accomplished when he surveyed the volume of work he had generated. We joked that the biggest single outcome of leukemia in our family was that we all worked hard and played hard all the time. Boredom was not a factor for us. In August, Catherine celebrated her long awaited tenth birthday with a swimming party, knowing that she was now ten years old and treatment would be over in the foreseeable future. It was a milestone.

In late August, we headed back out to Colorado for a week of riding and hiking. In addition to my sister and Danny, my mother joined us at the ranch. The cousins ran wild and their grandmother laughed at their antics and began to feel that she would survive the loss of her husband. Matthew at twelve was breaking away from the younger children and beginning to stick with the teenagers. David's sabbatical drew to a close and he confided to me that he had been afraid that if we were to lose Catherine, it would most likely happen during that year and he would need the time to be with her and Matt and me. It was the only time during the relapse that I remember him expressing his fear that she might die, although

I knew it was there as it was for all of us.

Matthew nervously headed off to junior high and Catherine, wearing her battery powered infusion pump, breezed into fifth grade. She was in a class with two teachers and 45 students and she was thrilled with them all. The alterations in her chemotherapy schedule allowed her to recuperate much more between doses of chemotherapy, so she seemed more well, more cheerful, and more enthusiastic about everything. We continued our interest in supporting the Charley Davidson Leukemia Fund. My video associates and I designed a public service announcement featuring Catherine which we hoped would raise money for research and patient amenities when it aired in the Christmas season. Catherine performed beautifully during the taping, requiring very few takes. She stated the case for support quite eloquently by saying, *There is a children's cancer clinic at the Massachusetts General Hospital. I know because I've been going there for six years.* All dressed in bright yellow, with her short pony tail tied in a ribbon, she looked so healthy it was almost shocking to hear her words.

On October 15, 1986, I gave another lecture at the junior high, this time to a class with Matthew in it. I worried about how he would tolerate his mother coming to teach about such a delicate subject. I need not have worried; he contributed a great deal of information, just as he did when he spoke to clinic groups. He told me later that I had done a pretty good job, which I took as high praise from our junior-high-aged son. Matthew still came to the clinic with us when he could. The clinic staff always treated him as a member of the team and he felt needed and respected there.

From Matt's college essays, 1991:

> *One time when Catherine was in remission, I was allowed by Sue, the nurse, to inject medicine into her small arm once the needle was in. It was a good feeling to be able to help Catherine in such a direct way, and this event reflected the trust that both she and Sue had in me.*

From the Journal, November 2, 1986:

> *Catherine gets the pump on Tuesday, hopefully for the last time. We are all getting excited and beginning to count the*

days until it is all over. Six long years in her short life. She is very nervous that we might have to do it all over again or worse. It is a strain for me to muster my own strength when she feels that way, but I do. Both children need my optimism and they are going to get it.

We were all working hard as Thanksgiving approached. Catherine and Matthew both made the honor roll in school, and David and I worked long days, frequently into the night, on writing projects, videos, and computer problems. My sister and Danny went to San Antonio while we took a whirlwind trip to Tulsa to see David's parents. His mother had been ill and she needed to see family. Seeing her son and grandchildren was uplifting for her. We were able to reassure her that Catherine was doing well. In early December, Catherine's public service announcement (PSA) began to run on three channels. It was a pleasure to see her sunny face on television. Occasionally someone from her school would see her and mention it, which made her feel good. The PSA drew attention to our clinic and was especially effective in getting clinic families to focus some of their energy toward raising funds for the clinic. My mother arrived for an extended Christmas visit and we all looked forward to the end of chemotherapy on December 30, 1986 when we would give Catherine her last dose of methotrexate and CCNU. She was scheduled for the last bone marrow and spinal tap on January 6, 1987.

We jumped with both feet into holiday preparations. The house was decorated from stem to stern and the tree was huge and filled with presents. The scout troop delivered bags of toys for the toy box and a toy manufacturer donated a large bag full of stuffed lambs, all of which we took to the clinic just as if we were Santa's helpers. The clinic ran Catherine's ad on their VCR whenever anyone mentioned it, and clearly we were all gearing up to celebrate her victory, or at least her survival to this point. Happily, Catherine tried out and was chosen for a part in the Children's Theater production of "Chitty Chitty, Bang Bang." She played the Baroness, an imperious, funny part, well suited to her.

Many people wondered at the time how we could keep from worrying about another relapse, especially given our previous experience. We did worry, all of us, each in his or her own way, but we just tried to keep it in perspective. Our celebrations all centered around surviving to this point in time and we were able to enjoy that victory.

From the Journal, December 27, 1986:

All things considered, 1986 will be a good year to see go by. It's been funny, sad, successful, and tragic, and we are ready for a new year. Catherine told me today that multiple relapses, when they happen, meant that a person can just be gone—just like that. She said that very directly and matter of factly. It is very sobering for a ten-year-old to talk like that.

30

Catherine Takes the Cake

A Boston television news magazine was planning a story on the Mass. General and they wanted to feature the Pediatric Hematology/Oncology Department as one segment of the program. They were planning on taping on January 6, the same day Catherine was scheduled for her final tests. We were called and asked if we would participate. While we preferred to stay out of the limelight in our day to day living, we believed it helpful to others to hear the clinic story and see the hope that comes from the families and staff. We agreed to the interview. We arrived at the clinic and Catherine talked to the TV people calmly about her illness and her experiences. When they found out that she was waiting for a bone marrow test they were surprised at her calm. The LP and bone marrow tests were done by Dr. Truman and went reasonably well. Catherine clutched the pillow, arched her back and started her methodical breathing, held her father's hand, and kept her gaze steady on her mother's face. At the conclusion of the tests we waited while Dr. Truman set up the slide and checked the microscope. Clear! After we heard the news, Catherine let the television crew return and she talked to them again. As we stood around smiling, Dr. Truman re-entered the treatment room with a cake to celebrate Catherine's big day. It was already after 5, dark outside, and very warm inside. We felt wonderful and Catherine sparkled with the attention. She was tremendously relieved to have the bone marrow test over! She had been working to live for six years and five months and now the hard part was over. We talked over what would happen next and learned that regular spinal taps would be performed at set intervals to catch any possible relapse at an early stage. We understood that the greatest risk was during the first year off treatment and that the risk decreased with time over a four year period, after which, with only a rare exception, she would be at no more risk than someone who had never had leukemia before.

From the medical records, January 6, 1987:

Completed chemotherapy! Looks wonderful. LP: clear. Bone Marrow: 0 Blasts. John Truman

From Catherine's letter to Helga, January, 1987:

Dear Helga, I have some very good news to tell you. On January 6, 1987, I got off my treatment for leukemia. It really made me feel great.

From the Journal, January 12, 1987:

Matthew and I just had a very good discussion about life and death and a lot of other stuff he had on his mind. Both of us enjoy the quiet time just before he falls asleep.

From a letter to Dr. Keefer, HCHP from Dr. Truman, January 15, 1987:

Catherine Krumme has finished her chemotherapy in grand style and her bone marrow and spinal fluid are normal. In fact, Channel 5 was in the clinic when she got the news of everything being normal and I hope it will be shown on Chronicle, January 17 at 7:30 p.m. We plan to check her monthly for the next year, then every 2 months for the year after, and then every 3 months.

As I told the TV cameras, I think her chance of outliving me is about 95%.

Many thanks and every best wish for the new year.

"Inside the Mass General," the one hour special done by Chronicle Magazine, aired on January 17, 1987. The program was excellent. Catherine was impressive and we enjoyed re-living the fact that the treatment was really over. The following month Catherine played the Baroness in the play and her friend Jason and his family sat prominently in the audience. Sue made a special trip to see Catherine in action. We are always especially touched by interaction with our clinic friends.

From a clinic mother, April, 1987:

> *Dear Cynthia, I saw you and Catherine on television—Chronicle—and I was so happy to see you celebrate that special day. I have thought of you often. Our lives are back on track now, but it has taken a long time since our son's death in 1981.*

From Catherine's medical record, April 28, 1987:

> *Catherine looks wonderful! With each visit off chemotherapy, she looks better and better! Sue Thompson.*

For the next year, Catherine was given periodic spinal taps. Because they were less frequent, she lost some of her trained and practiced ability to focus away from the pain, but she held still and endured. We tried to renew friendships that had waited during the years of intensive chemotherapy when we lived our lives completely on clinic time, and we adjusted to the growing separation between our family and our clinic family. Dr. Truman left the clinic for new work and Dr. Ferguson took charge. Dr. Robbins came back from France and Monica stayed the same as always. Sue was back working full time at the clinic. We traveled during the summer to Scandinavia and to Iceland to visit Catherine's friend Helga, and we went hiking again in Colorado. We relished the fact that for the first time in three years we could be gone from Massachusetts for more than two weeks because we didn't have such frequent clinic responsibilities. Catherine entered the sixth grade and Matt the eighth. She tried out again for the Children's Theater production and earned a wonderful part as the TV announcer in "Willy Wonka and the Chocolate Factory." Jason made the trip again with his family, this time just after another relapse. He greeted Catherine enthusiastically and made her day. The toy box was filled again by the local scouts and our clinic visits became less and less frequent. Now that Catherine was more of a social visitor there, we no longer knew everything that was happening and we missed many aspects of that knowledge. We still suffered the sorrows of losing our friends when their illness proved stronger than the treatment, but we missed the warmth of frequent contact with people who knew us so well. Most clinic families miss the people for a long time after they leave the clinic.

Despite the fact that our clinic visits were infrequent, the subject of leukemia came up more and more often as the children grew older and their abilities to comprehend the disease became more sophisticated. Every clinic visit brought hours of discussion. In the winter of 1987, Matt wrote a short story called "Joe" about two teenage friends, one of whom developed leukemia and struggled to survive. His story won a certificate of achievement from the Read Writing Awards Program. David and I began to realize the extent of the impact of the cancer experience on our children. We had always worried that their experiences would hurt them so much that their lives would not be happy and that their futures would be adversely impacted, but instead of being defeated and beaten, they have emerged as strong, sensitive individuals who walk through their lives with optimism and joy. We have learned how resilient human beings are.

From the Journal, January 2, 1988:

> *Two more children have died and we are shaken. The clinic world is a world unto itself where life and death ride side by side on a roller coaster that never stops. Who lives and who dies seems completely arbitrary and without rhyme or reason. The riders and their families don't know which seat to take and it is a matter of luck at every turn.*

1988 began with the death from an infection of my youngest sister Rebecca. She became sick on January 2nd and died on the 3rd. We were stunned. I went to Oklahoma to make arrangements for her and while I was away Matt became ill with a fever. One week later, I was home and he was worse. He was finally diagnosed with osteomyelitis, a bacterial bone infection, in his left upper leg. He spent 12 days hospitalized in the Mass. General on high doses of antibiotics. Having Matt in the hospital was devastating for Catherine. She felt it was acceptable if she had to go, but not her brother! Matt's infection responded to antibiotics, and within two or three days he was at least feeling better. He was an agreeable patient, helped by frequent visits from his family, school friends, and, much to his delight, all the doctors and nurses from Catherine's clinic. David and I were relieved that a diagnosis had been made and that the disease was curable. We just couldn't believe our "healthy child" had become so sick. Several of the floor nurses we had known when Catherine was hospitalized also took care of Matt. While they were sorry he was ill, they all expressed relief that the Krumme on the admissions list was not Catherine. While hospitalized, Matt heard that a fourteen-year-old girl newly diagnosed with leukemia was in a room up the hall. Using crutches and pushing his IV pole, he went to visit her, telling her she must keep fighting and keep up her spirits. He made quite an impression during his stay at the MGH, and the experience made a lasting impression on him as well.

From Matt's college essays, 1991:

I have learned empathy for people in difficult circumstances, as well as an awareness of the strengths people exhibit in fighting to stay alive. I have tried to share my experience with others by giving talks to medical personnel and others who were interested. At one point I had a chance to see what hospital life was like when I was diagnosed with osteomyelitis and spent many days in the hospital. There I introduced myself to a girl my age who had just been diagnosed with leukemia, and I was able to relate to her some of my sister's experiences and be as supportive as I could. I also went through treatment of my own in that period. It was enlightening to become a host for so many needles and the subject of so many doctors, and the experience increased my appreciation for what Catherine went through.

From the Journal, January 19, 1988:

Catherine is very weepy about Matthew's illness. She is somewhat overwhelmed by the events and by the fact that he could be sick. We are all rather out of sorts. This has been a tragic time.

31

It's Over?

We had anticipated that getting used to being off treatment would take time for all of us. We had not anticipated how long it would take to get back to normal. Catherine had been ill for so long that we couldn't remember what normal might even be. When stresses and strains of loss and change occurred in other parts of our lives we knew we were still reacting as we had during the treatment years. We had become stoic. Catherine took Bactrim prophylactically for the first year. Her hair, which had been slowly growing in since 1985, was still thin and not what she remembered from pre-leukemia days. We noticed that her strength and endurance improved by leaps and bounds, but she did not always recognize that fact. Her self image needed work.

From the Journal, February 5, 1988:

> *Catherine had another crying jag this morning. She feels badly about her hair, her status, her friends, in short about everything. Usually it is her hair that sets her off. I think her self image needs work and we plan to address those issues. Matthew is trying to help her by telling her she is special, cute, funny, etc. He is very thoughtful.*

Once Catherine was finished with chemotherapy, we actually breathed a collective sigh of relief. The chemotherapy during the relapse years was so strenuous that we were often under considerable strain. Of course, after treatment ended we were well aware of the possibility of a relapse; however, we were not plagued by fear of one. After the first year the chances of relapse diminished as they did during each subsequent year. We all put on a brave face to the world, although concerns would occasionally slip through to the surface. From the Journal, April 4, 1988:

> *Catherine stayed home today due to illness. I have not handled it well. It is difficult not to become fearful when she complains of fatigue and aching bones. The fact that she also has cold symptoms is reassuring.*

From the Winchester Star, May 26, 1988:

> *A real winner, in my opinion, is a young sixth-grade soccer player named Catherine Krumme. Catherine has been playing soccer for years, and she's a good little player. But often she has played when she's been sick, as Catherine has been fighting cancer for more that half of her young life. She is well now, and it's such a joy to watch her being a regular kid. The courage and determination which pulled her through the tough years should be an inspiration to all. Her type of "winning" is the win that really counts.*

A few days after the article appeared our phone rang and both Matt and Catherine picked it up. I heard Matt scream, *Catherine, hang up!* and I went running. The voice on the phone had said, *I wish you had died from leukemia.* Our experience is not atypical of people who become well known, but it has been shocking that a child could be subjected to such treatment. As a result of that event we felt it best for her to keep a low profile, although we continued to believe that there was a value in others seeing a child with cancer succeed in normal ways. We continued to participate in talks to medical people and patients, but we avoided mentioning cancer around our town.

Catherine's sixth grade teacher and her principal wanted to give her a special gift at her graduation and congratulate her publicly for the accomplishment of doing well and graduating with her class in spite of having leukemia throughout her elementary school career. After careful consideration we asked that they not do anything publicly because of the phone experience and because Catherine was being teased at school for *acting like a grown-up* and was struggling to find a place for herself. She did not want to be publicly noticed by anyone in authority at school. Her teacher privately gave her a lovely graduation necklace which she treasures.

In October 1988, as a seventh grader, Catherine was given a merit award by a panel of teachers and students for being conscientious, responsible, cheerful, and heroic. The principal said, *She always has a positive attitude and is an inspiration to us all.* When the award was announced, several other students told her she didn't deserve it and asked her what made her so special anyway. Catherine's fighting spirit came the closest it ever has to collapsing during those times. She indicated that she would like to forget cancer completely and we tried to help her. Not until ninth grade did Catherine feel that she would like to give talks again. She has resumed doing so and feels good about the decision. She now occasionally mentions that she had leukemia to someone in much the same way one would discuss a broken leg or a trip. Her hair is a little thin and that bothers her, but she is strong and healthy and she knows it. The fact that Catherine was in junior high during this stressful period is probably part of the explanation for the problems we experienced. It is a difficult time for many young people and they all seem to have problems dealing with being different in any way. In her case, it was a bad time for a person who had already seen a lot tough times.

From the Coordinator, Parent-Child Nursing Program, Boston University:

> *Dear Catherine, On behalf of the students and the teachers in the School of Nursing, I wish to thank you for your willingness to come to class and talk with the nurses. You shared with us many of the important things we should know about children and cancer and we all learned a great deal.*

Catherine received diagnostic spinal taps until September, 1988. Since the end of chemotherapy there had been no replacement fluid used in the taps, and the loss of spinal fluid caused spinal headaches. She was highly susceptible to them and usually had a severe headache for several days after the tap. We tried everything in an attempt to minimize them, but the headaches were always a problem. Dr. Ferguson began taking only the most minute amount of fluid that could be diagnostic and even then the headaches were severe. The end of the spinal taps was a time for celebration. Catherine felt she had passed a major hurdle.

From the medical records, September 20, 1988:

Catherine has been great. She had a wonderful summer. No problems since her last visit. It has been eight years since diagnosis. Diagnostic LP: clear. Sue Thompson

From the Journal, September 27, 1988:

Last week, Catherine had what we hope was her last spinal tap ever. It went smoothly with her friend Jason lying on the bed next to hers getting his chemo. For him it just goes on and on; he is a brave child.

Catherine has grown into a lovely, happy, young woman. Though she has had some stressful moments, her development is normal, she does well in school, and she has a pleasant, friendly disposition. She and her brother are close. The clinic experience will stay with her as it will with her family. It doesn't haunt her, it is just part of her life. She keeps in touch with Sue, who has left the clinic, married, and had a little girl of her own. Catherine did one of the readings at Sue's wedding in Ohio and Lauren's parents joined us there. It was a day of celebration.

From the Journal, October, 1989:

The wedding was lovely. Louise and Bob were a sight for sore eyes. They remain as wonderful as ever. Catherine danced with Bob and Louise and I loved it. This is my fifth journal volume since 1980. Lauren has figured in the last three. It is fitting that she is still with us. She would have loved the dancing.

Epilogue

We still visit the clinic twice a year for a blood test and a social visit. Since Catherine absorbed more total chemotherapy than just about anyone else who survived, the doctors are especially interested in looking for long term side-effects, of which there have been few. The cub scouts from our town are still filling the toy box as they have for the last eight years. Our loyal friend Jason lost his battle in early 1991 and his mother held Catherine long and tightly at his wake. Scores of clinic friends are off treatment and healthy. Of the five local children we knew with leukemia, all have survived.

From Matt's college essays, 1991:

Now, as Catherine is completely cured and a sophomore in high school, I rarely think about the fact that she spent so much of her life being sick, but what I learned and gained from this ordeal stays with me. I may not yet realize all the ways in which I have been affected, but I think my sensitivity and the need I feel to help people who are sick, upset, or vulnerable are definitely the outcome of years of growing up with a sister with leukemia.

In December 1991, the MGH Newsletter featured an article about Catherine which talked about her experiences, her clinic rules, and her positive attitude. It was entitled "Sitting on Top of the World" and featured a photo of her sitting at the summit of Long's Peak, the climb she made unassisted two days before her 15th birthday. Hope rolled off the pages of the article, just as it has been a force in our lives for over twelve years.

From the MGH Newsletter, by Linda Goodspeed, December 1991:

Cynthia Krumme

Catherine has been off treatment now for four years and four months. With every passing month the chances of her leukemia remaining in remission improve. "The general feeling now is that if a child's leukemia remains in remission seven years, the chances of the leukemia coming back are extremely small—not zero—but extremely small," Dr. Ferguson said. "It's always nice to see kids years off treatment coming back to visit with their own kids in tow. It's something that 20 years ago, no one would have dared hope or think. Now we see it all the time."

Catherine, December, 1991:

Children with cancer must have a strong will in order to survive. They must be more determined, braver, and stronger than their peers. They must learn to take every needle and pill in stride, viewing each as just another challenge set before them. Depression and feeling sorry for oneself are pits that are easy to fall into unless one is very careful. Hope and optimism are essential.

Give the Gift of Hope to Your Friends and Colleagues!

ORDER FORM

YES, I want ___ copies of *Having Leukemia Isn't So Bad. Of Course It Wouldn't Be My First Choice* at $9.95 each, plus $3 shipping per book. (Massachusetts residents please include $.50 state sales tax.) Canadian orders must be accompanied by a postal money order in U.S. funds.

___ Check/money order enclosed ★ Charge my ___ VISA ___ MC

Name _____ Phone _____

Organization _____

Address _____

City/State/Zip _____

Card # _____ Expires _____

Signature _____

Call your credit card order to:
(617) 729-9037

Please make your check payable and return to:
Sargasso Enterprises
14 Wildwood Street
Winchester, MA 01890